Introduction to Karate-Dō

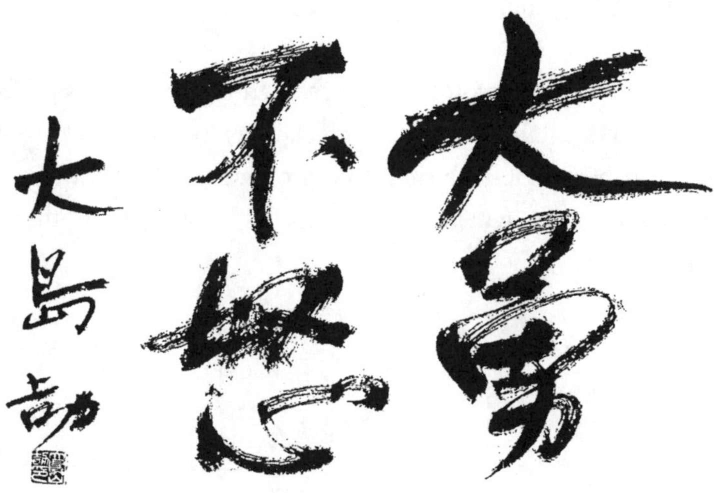

A Study Guide for Beginning Students of Shotokan — Ohshima Karate

Michael Mantz
Tom Muzila

Pine Winds Press
An imprint of Idyll Arbor, Inc.
39129 264th Ave SE, Enumclaw, WA 98022
www.PineWindsPress.com

Pine Winds Press Editor: Thomas M. Blaschko

Calligraphy by Tsutomu Ohshima
Translation: A truly valiant mind is not easily irritated.
(A courageous man is not easily drawn into a fight.)

ISBN 9780937663301

To my wife Elva Mantz, whose support has been unconditional.

In memory of Don DePree.

Shotokan Karate of America
Mission Statement

The mission of Shotokan Karate of America, as established by its Shihan, Tsutomu Ohshima, is to "preserve, perpetuate, and advance the legacy of Shotokan Karate for the betterment of the lives of those who train, and to contribute positively to human history."

米國松濤館

Contents

Foreword

We all start karate practice for various reasons — to learn self-defense, for involvement in the sporting aspect, and/or for the excellent overall exercise it presents — but this outstanding book goes beyond that. It lays a solid foundation which starts each student on the transcendent path of karate-dō — karate as a "way of life" — which is the essence of our practice!

With this book, Michael Mantz, an outstanding practitioner and instructor of karate-dō, challenges students in ways that, with practice, will help them better their lives through training, which in turn, one student at a time, will help to better society and, thus, humanity itself. I hope this understanding, along with this book's guidance, will stimulate each student to make the practice truly relevant, by bringing its ideals into his or her daily life. In the words of Master Funakoshi, "When you look at life, think in terms of karate. But remember that karate is not only karate; it is life."

Don DePree
Godan, Shotokan Karate of America

Preface

The most important and toughest opponent a karate person or martial artist can face is himself or herself. You must face your weaknesses, fears, insecurities, and mental blocks. When you face an extremely strong opponent, or situation in life, these mental blocks will be exposed, first from your subconscious mind. In karate, we call this, to polish or cut oneself first. This means to criticize and judge yourself before you judge others. Michael Mantz has practiced this concept his entire life. He has integrated it with teaching karate and his lectures. He has polished every aspect of his mind at the deepest extent. This character and integrity will be exposed in the information of this book.

The book is focused toward the beginning student. All the information will educate you on important facets related to a good, strong understanding of karate's fundamental foundation. The book is written in a very comprehensive way. It will educate you to many deeper elements of karate's true nature. You will learn not only about the practice and training of karate, but also concepts of how you can use it to benefit and supplement your life experiences. These principles can be directly applicable to a more successful life. The contents of this book will cover basic history, how to acquire the proper attitude toward practice, and karate's foundational structure. Proper forms of the hand, striking, kicking, and blocking will be addressed. Forms (katas) and sparring or fighting (kumite) will be explained.

There are questions, answers, and definitions in the back of the book, which you will easily be able to learn. You will acquire a broad spectrum of knowledge about karate. This will give you a great foundation to initiate your practice with the proper attitude and mentality.

Tom Muzila
Godan, Shotokan Karate of America

Briefly I would like to thank the many Shotokan Karate of America seniors who have helped me to develop my own practice and understanding by their direct or indirect guidance. Their level and their knowledge humbles my own. There are so many to mention, the list would be long. I would however like to recognize just a few, Tom Muzila, Jim Sagawa, Don DePree, Kei Teramoto, and my original senior Frank Flores. These seniors and many more, have been an inspiration with their positive encouragement and direction. My sincere gratitude goes out to them for teaching me to always push myself and to clearly face myself in practice and in life.

To my seniors, I also ask for their patience and to forgive me if I have not articulated some of the concepts clearly or if I have inadvertently excluded some key principles.

To my juniors, thank you for being a mirror of my ability to "pass on the way." Please continue to practice and to improve on what you have begun.

Lastly, I would be remiss if I didn't mention Master Tsutomu Ohshima, the Shihan and founder of Shotokan Karate of America and many international karate groups (including groups in Canada, Israel, France, Morocco, and many others).

Ohshima Sensei has literally given his life to spread karate-dō throughout the entire globe, illuminating many peoples from many ethnic and political backgrounds to the fundamental teachings of Master Funakoshi and karate-dō. He has unselfishly sacrificed himself in this endeavor. Tom Muzila in his book *Mental Karate: A Warrior's Guide* states, "There are very few people on the planet who are the total embodiment of a warrior saint. Tsutomu Ohshima is one of those rare souls and human beings. The essence of the ancient warrior would not exist to the degree it does today if it were not for his life and teachings."[1]

Ohshima Sensei is what the ancient Tao, Confucian, and Buddhist traditions called the "superior man." Zen masters would call him "a true man of no title."

Ohshima Sensei is truly one of those rare individuals who comes along once every century. He is a true master and an enlightened human being. I am honored to know him and to have received his instruction and guidance.

I thank Ohshima Sensei for his teachings, for his leadership, and for his many letters of encouragement over the last thirty-five years.

Thank-you, Ohshima Sensei for your support which has enabled me to develop this small book.

Rev. Deacon Michael Mantz
Shotokan Karate of America, Corpus Christi Dōjō

---

[1] Tom Muzila, *Mental Karate*, p. 12.

Acknowledgments

I would humbly like to thank Tom Muzila for sharing his insights on karate-dō with me and for his continued guidance and support for many years. Thank you to my wife Elva Mantz for her many hours of typing and editing.

A special acknowledgement is given to the following individuals for their contributions:

- Photographs — April Martinez Ocañas, Jonathan R. Kanick
- Illustrations — Thermon Biggers, Virginia Monsibais
- Maps and History Chart — Robert Patrick Cenci

I would like to thank my juniors who posed for the photographs: Steven Flores, Bethany Hood, and Alex Shurin.

Thank you to my senior Don DePree for granting permission to reference his practice notes and use his photos.

Lastly, to Ohshima Sensei for giving his permission and for his encouragement.

Introduction

It is important to look at what we are doing in training, to think about the real reason why we practice. In Japanese, the word is keiko. The character "kei" means to think and "ko" means old or ancient. So practice, keiko, means to think of the ancient, that is to think back to the masters.

When we practice, this is what we do. We try to understand the lessons the masters of the past has transmitted to us through the katas (forms) and more recently through the basics and methods of sparring described by Master Funakoshi.[1]

Tsutomu Ohshima
Shihan, Shotokan Karate of America

This small book is an accumulation of my own training in Shotokan Karate — Ohshima for over thirty-five years and in teaching a college credit course since 1983. It is also in collaboration with my senior, Tom Muzila, who helped me co-author this work with his insights, guidance, and understanding of the training concepts of karate-dō. I thank him for helping me to develop my own karate level, and for laying the foundations for the Special Trainings that have been held in Corpus Christi, Texas, in conjunction with Shotokan Karate of America.

My personal knowledge (as an adjunct professor) in presenting karate-dō as a university kinesiology credit course has enabled me to know what really works and what does not, in terms of the student's comprehension of the subject matter (given the short, three and a half month timeframe for a college credit course).

Karate-dō, however, is not something that can be experienced in a brief college-semester setting. As the title of the publication states, this is an “introduction,” with the underlying meaning that it barely scratches the surface.

To the senior practitioner, the concepts covered in this work will probably seem rudimentary. For beginners, however, I hope you will find the chapters in this book helpful in augmenting your understanding of the foundational core movements that are requisite to the course structure.

We as humans are very complex beings. We are a unique blend of mental, emotional, spiritual, and physical beings. This work will stress the physical but will also touch on those other aspects of our human personhood and how they relate to our karate training. It is no secret that in order to reach any level of success, our practice and development must contain all of these aspects working simultaneously and in harmony. But to arrive at this point, we must first dedicate ourselves to practicing wholeheartedly the physical techniques of karate.

The major focus of this publication will be to create a foundation on which we can build a powerful structure. The theory being, once we have a strong base, we can stack many levels of understanding on top without toppling the structure. However, if our base is weak or flawed in some way, the resulting layered structure will eventually crumble. I once observed a 25-story office tower being constructed from the vantage point of my nearby office window.

I was amazed to see how long it took to complete the foundation of this structure. It seemed like the steam shovels would excavate forever. After the completion of this huge pit in the ground, the foundation was then fitted and piled with steel beams. There seemed to be no end to the huge trucks that kept pouring concrete, which framed and encased the steel reinforcement pilings. Once the foundation was complete, the superstructure itself seemed to be erected rather quickly. This structure is very well built and stands solid today after many years of serving thousands of people every day. It stands very proud, very tall, and very strong on its solid foundation, just as karate students seek to erect a strong level of understanding based on their solid karate foundation.

The practice of karate-dō is very similar to the example of the building in that we must first build a strong foundation — a foundation that will allow us to build many layers of understanding without having it crumble. Just as men construct a building with its foundation or nature constructs a tree with strong roots, the karate student must also construct his or her root system or foundation.

Our prime objective, therefore, with this book and the accompanying course will be to build core values and the foundational structure of the karate "pyramid." To illustrate this concept of foundation, as it relates to your karate practice, I would like to use a diagram created by Tom Muzila that delineates the different traditional karate levels of black belt and the corresponding developmental understanding in the areas of physical, spiritual, and mental awareness. Mr. Muzila graphically displays this understanding of Master Tsutomu Ohshima with the pyramid structure shown on the next page.

Notice the bottom level of the pyramid structure. It is wide and solid. The structure is very well balanced and firmly rooted. This same principle can be applied to anything that we are trying to perfect as a human endeavor. Once we create a base that is strong and solid, we can build many things on top, knowing that our foundation will support the built-up structure.

The pyramid illustration can be even further expanded by adding the stages of development prior to the first black belt level.

The wavy line drawn across the bottom of the third black belt level is similar to the level of water around an iceberg. We know that the majority of the massive iceberg structure is hidden below the surface of the water. Similarly, a skilled martial artist who seemingly has a smooth, powerful technique (on the surface) is someone who has developed the foundation of their art for many years which enables the body, conscious mind, and unconscious mind to move as one single unit.

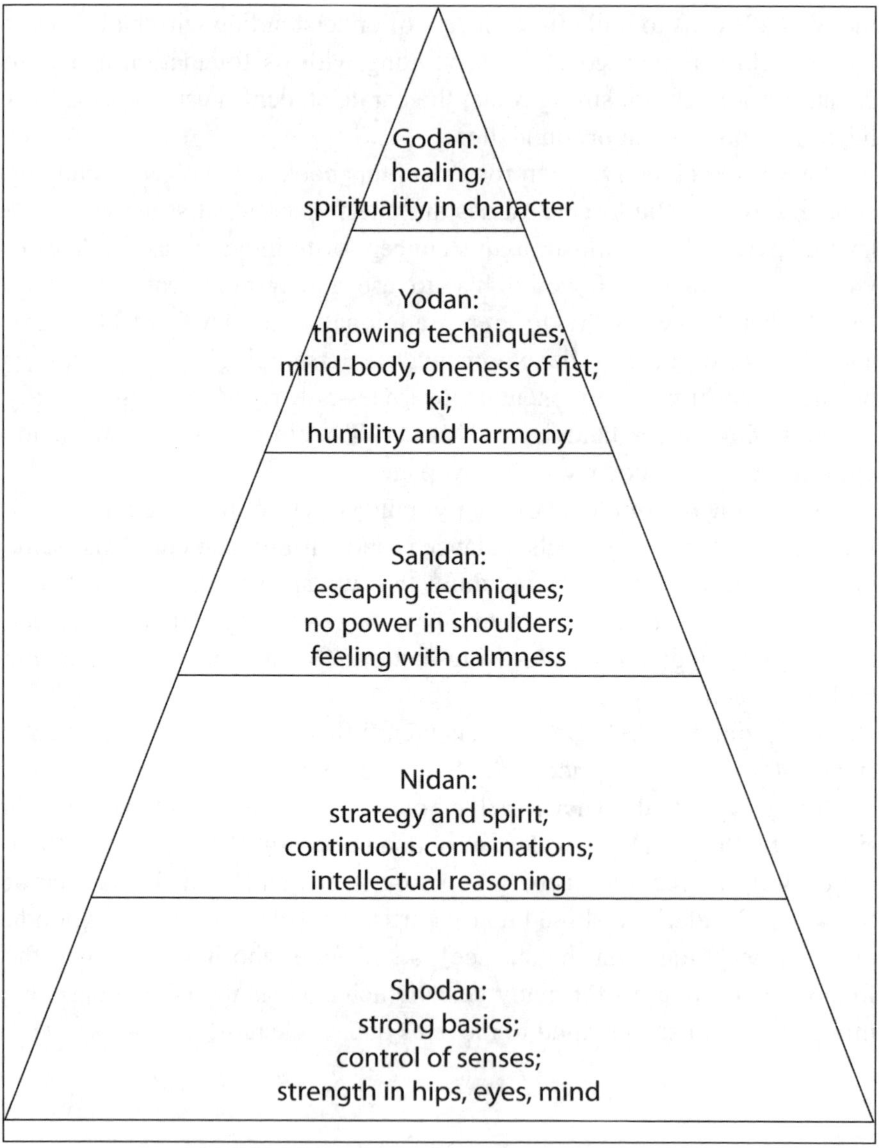

Figure 1: Shotokan Karate of America attributes or understandings that accompany black belt levels. (Ohshima Sensei and Tom Muzila)

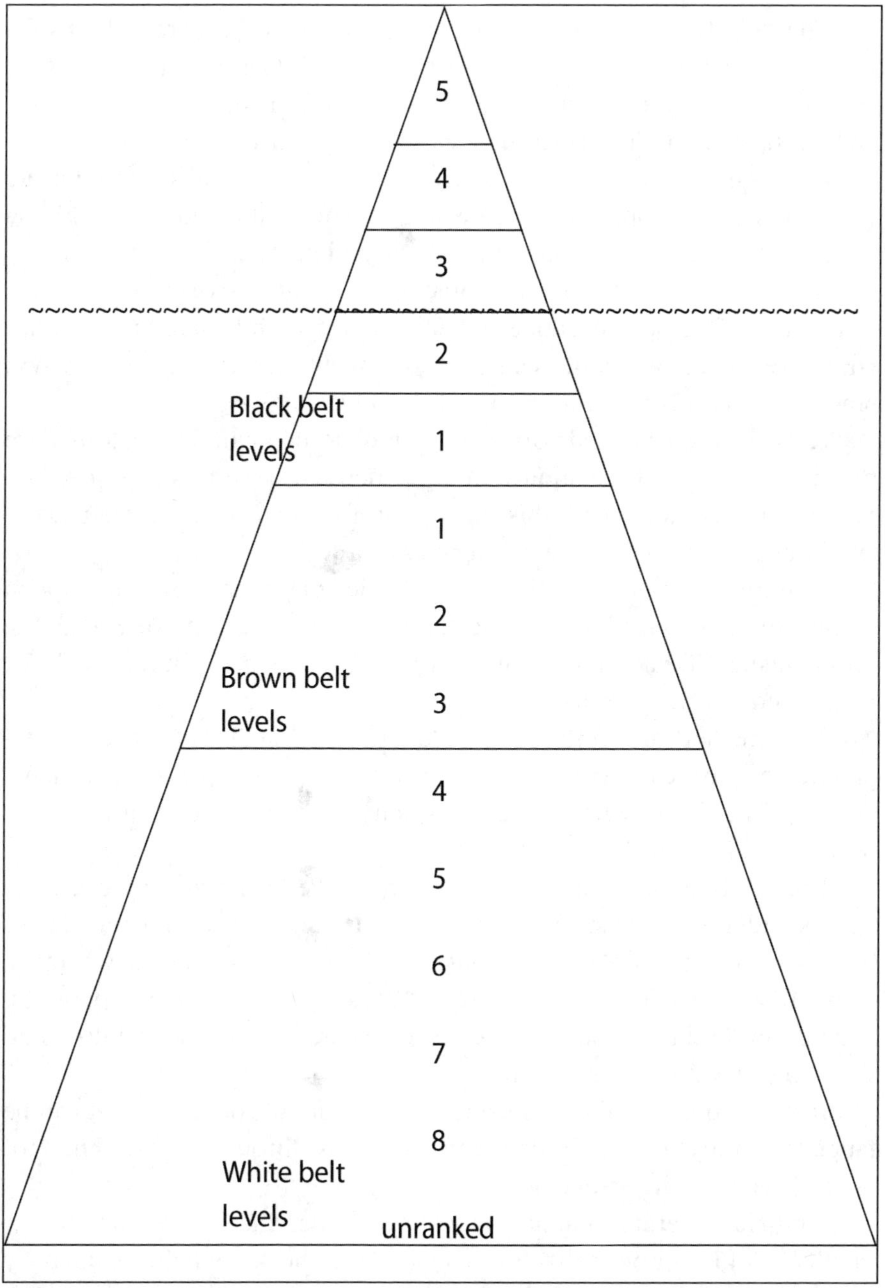

Figure 2: Pyramid showing all levels. (Michael Mantz)

The "hidden" foundation is what I refer to as the core values of a karate practitioner. These core values can be divided into the following concepts: techniques, stances, eyes, hips, power lines, pulling hand, underarm, standing leg, breathing, and fighting spirit.

Consequently, the desired objective of our class will be to dedicate our efforts in developing these core values. This will be done through the three major facets of practice: kihon, kata, and kumite.

Kihon — The one by one practicing of offensive and defensive techniques. This will be done either in place or by marching forward with a series of the same technique one technique at a time. We will practice thousands of techniques in this way during class.

Kata — Pre-arranged forms that simulate combat. These forms are practiced with exact techniques in a geometrical pattern and set rhythm. Seven katas are shown in this book. The first two or three are usually taught in a one-semester, beginning class.

Kumite — Sparring (combat). Basic one-time sparring (ippon gumite) will be introduced, using the sparring kata, Ten No Kata, as a pre-requisite. Basic three-time sparring (sanbon gumite) will be introduced as time permits.

The method of building our karate base will be presented by practicing physical repetitions of a learned technique (kihon, kata, kumite). This is known as developing muscle memory to ensure that we initially learn the techniques properly.

I prefer to explain this concept of repetitive techniques by using the understanding of Master Tsutomu Ohshima, the shihan and founder of Shotokan Karate of America. Ohshima Sensei says that as we make many repetitions of our techniques, "We begin to train our powerful unconscious mind, which is directly connected to our conscious mind through our method of breathing."[2]

In short, our techniques become part of our subconscious that can be tapped into by our everyday consciousness through our method of breathing and bodily movements.

Authentic karate practice is always experienced. No amount of intellect, logic, or verbalization can replace the knowledge gained by your own sweat and determination. Karate must be practiced in such a way, that our kihon, kata, and kumite always relate back to an opponent.

In other words, our practice must be realistic, not idealistic. This is a self-defense and combat art. So, in a sense, we have to become people who understand combat and combat situations. Others can help guide us by using their own expertise to teach and move us along, but we ourselves must be our own lamps, lighting our own way along the path. To illustrate this concept, there is a story told by Goso Hōyen of the 12th-century Chinese Sung dynasty. The following short story illustrates the Zen spirit that goes beyond intellect, logic, and words.[3]

> If people ask me what Zen is like I will say that it is like learning the art of burglary. The son of a burglar saw his father growing older and thought, "If he is unable to carry on his profession, who will be the bread winner of the family, except for myself? I must learn the trade." He intimated the idea to his father who approved of it.
>
> One night the father took the son to a big house, broke through the fence, entered the house, and, opening one of the large chests, told the son to go in and pick out the clothing. As soon as the son got into it, the father dropped the lid and securely applied the lock. The father now came out to the court-yard and loudly knocked at the door, waking up the family; then he slipped away by the hole in the fence. The residents got excited and lighted candles but they found that the burglar had already gone.
>
> The son who had remained all the time securely confined in the chest thought of his cruel father. He was greatly mortified, then a fine idea flashed upon him. He made a noise like the gnawing of a rat. The family told the maid to take a candle and examine the chest.
>
> When the lid was unlocked, out came the prisoner, who blew out the light, pushed away from the maid, and fled. The people ran after him. Noticing a well by the road he picked up a large stone and threw it into the water. The pursuers all gathered around the well trying to find the burglar drowning himself in the dark hole.

> In the meantime, he went safely back to his father's house and blamed him deeply for his narrow escape. Said the father, "Be not offended my son. Just tell me how you got out of it." When the son told him all about his adventures, the father remarked, "There you are, you have learned the art."
>
> The idea of the story demonstrates the futility of verbal instruction and conceptual presentation as far as the experience of enlightenment is concerned.
>
> Understanding must be the out growth of one's inner life and experience, and not a verbal implantation brought from the outside.
>
> The Tao ("ultimate reality" or "truth") as stated by Mencius (the great Chinese Confucian scholar), is near, and people seek it far away. This means, that the Tao is our everyday life itself.

In relation gaining an understanding in karate-dō, it simply means that we ourselves must experience the struggles of going through the knothole. We ourselves must experience how it feels, as opposed to having someone tell us how it is supposed to feel. Someone can tell you what it feels like to face a strong opponent, but you will never learn about it, until you have faced that situation (and not just a single time, but many times).

"Fugu kuwanu hito niwa iwaji". ("It is impossible to describe the taste of blowfish to one who has never eaten it.")[4] This Japanese proverb stated by Master Funakoshi gives further meaning to what has been related above. Similarly, the true nature of karate-dō cannot be explained in words even if one's efforts with pen or tongue are carried to the point of exhaustion and beyond.

Keeping this in mind I hope that this small book will help to augment and clarify your practice of traditional karate-dō. This work will also cite *Karate-Dō Kyōhan: The Master Text* by Gichin Funakoshi (translated by Tsutomu Ohshima) as a suggested reference text. Each chapter will conclude with suggested reading. This heading will direct the student to the chapter(s) in the *Kyōhan*, which will help to clarify and elucidate the material being presented.

The chapters in this work are summarized in the following manner:

The next section, entitled Karate-Dō describes Ohshima Sensei's view on karate as a part of Budō.

Chapter 1 contains a summary of the history and development of karate-dō. This is not an attempt on my part to make any clearer what has already been recorded by the many great karate masters (including Master Funakoshi). It is simply presented to give you a historical perspective on how this noble martial art went from the indigenous Okinawan method of self-defense that was influenced by the Chinese experts to the "Way of the Empty Hand" that we recognize today. This discussion will include the *Bubishi* (Bible of Karate) and the major experts (Chinese, Okinawan, and Japanese) who helped to develop and spread the art of karate in Okinawa, Japan, and the United States.

Chapter 2 consists of a basic introduction to the formalities of traditional karate practice.

Chapter 3 delineates the core foundational concepts of our practice.

Chapter 4 covers the basic hand techniques.

Chapter 5 covers the basic foot techniques.

Chapter 6 covers seven basic katas.

Chapter 7 introduces the basic types of sparring practice.

Chapter 8 contains some further thoughts on the concepts and principals of practicing karate-dō.

---

[1] Tsutomu Ohshima, *Notes on Training*, pp. 1-2.
[2] *Ibid.*, pp. 215-216.
[3] D.T. Suzuki, *Zen and Japanese Culture*, pp. 9-10.
[4] Gichin Funakoshi, *Karate-Dō Nyūmon*, p. 12.

Karate-Dō

Master Tsutomu Ohshima is the Shihan and founder of Shotokan Karate of America. His meditation on karate-dō, shown below, is one of the finest insights on the subject. As you work through this book, I encourage you to continually return to this meditation for that is what it truly is, a meditation. The more you practice, the more insight you will have when you revisit this profound reflection.

This was written by Master Tsutomu Ohshima in August 1981 for the twenty-fifth anniversary of the start of Nisei Week in Los Angeles.[1]

> Having taught karate here since my arrival as a foreign student in 1955, I have come to believe that American society truly possesses an amazing energy and great generosity.
>
> I have wondered why the people of a nation which emerged victorious in World War II showed interest in the culture of the defeated nation of Japan, especially in karate, which is an element of ancient Budō. While seeking an answer to this question, I have been given the opportunity to continue to practice karate, and through it I have been able to affirm my own attitude towards life.
>
> What is Budō? Bujutsu seeks out methods to defeat an opponent on the battlefield. Budō, however, begins with the concept of "one's cutting of oneself" (onore a kiru). In other words, in Budō we realize that one's true opponent is oneself, and in constantly trying to imagine ourselves in the face of death, we seek to forge, harden, and discipline our minds and bodies. In this manner we try to push on to utmost limits of our strength.

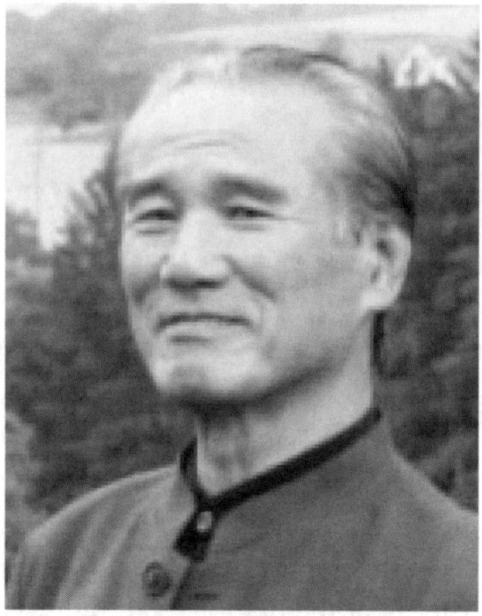

Master Tsutomu Ohshima

This is not the final goal of practice, though. What we seek through such training is to unshackle ourselves from external pressure and oppression and be truly free in will and action. Philosophically speaking, Budō strives to make the leap from the relative to the absolute; and thus rising above the violence of the battlefield, it points the way to peace and harmony.

In other Oriental training methods whose goal is to heighten mental awareness, there is a dependence on books or on consciously moving the body or consciously controlling breathing. Budō, however, stresses the importance of actual experience and training of the unconscious mind. For this reason, as much as possible, Budō avoids intellectual knowledge gained through words or sentences. Instead it stresses the union of mind, body, and breathing while facing an opponent, especially in life-or-death situations.

To always face one's opponent directly means to face death directly. Budō demands the energy, spirit, and strength necessary to criticize oneself strictly and honestly. Thus, through facing death every day, we can come to understand the difficulties we face in our daily lives; and through the daily practice of karate, we become able to cast away anger and fear. In this way, we can come to appreciate the value of an even, temperate mind (heijo shin).

The practice of Budō knows no boundaries of East and West, and recognizes no differences as to race or nationality. Someday in the near future, the essential concepts of Budō will become a part of the vocabulary of all languages. For example, those who are training in America have no problem in understanding the significance of "removing power from the shoulders" (kata no chikara o nuku), "lowering the hips" (koshi o otosu), "getting the right breathing" (kokyu o taitoku suru) or "the sense of ma" (ma no kankaku).

The practice of Budō will have great significance in the building of a new society in which, unlike the twentieth century where a man is evaluated by his wealth, new standards will be the strength, purity, warmth, and richness of the mind.

Furthermore, the human relationships of master and disciple, and of senior and junior, so important to Budō, will come to play a significant role in future society. Such relationships must be based on the realization that only one's example can help others push themselves. Then the senior can lead his juniors with a warm heart, and the junior can respect his senior and follow him. In such a relationship, each must consider that he has three lives: his senior's life, his own, and that of junior. I see such relationships forming the vertical threads that will interweave as a fabric with the horizontal, democratic structure of Western society. The emerging material, representing the qualitative changes of advancement in the evolution of the human spirit, will contribute to the creation of a new tapestry for future generations. Dō means a "way" or "precept" that can be positively proved through experience. Budō's fate and true nature lies in the recognition and absolute affirmation of one's gains through experience. In striving to face one's opponent and one's death without deviation, there is no room for false or empty philosophy.

This is the basis for my belief that Budō has the quality to ensure it a place in world vocabulary. Relying on this belief and harboring no feeling of doubt, I have continued to practice for the past twenty-five years with the young people of the world.

---

[1] From Tsutomu Ohshima. (1998). Notes on Training. Enumclaw, WA: Pine Winds Press.

1.
History of Karate-Dō

Personally, I think that Ryūkyū kempō in other words karate, originated as an indigenous Okinawan martial art. In periods when Chinese culture was held in high esteem, practitioners went abroad to learn Chinese martial arts, adding to their native Okinawan methods or te. Through comparative research the best elements were selected and the character kara [empty hand] was adopted. Thus, I feel that what is known today as karate has a rich, wholesome history of development.[1]

Gichin Funakoshi

Master Gichin Funakoshi, in his book, *Karate-Dō: My Way of Life*, relates that the history of how or when karate was introduced to the Ryūkyūs is clouded and uncertain.[2] (The Ryūkyūs are a chain of islands stretching from southern Japan to Taiwan, including Okinawa). This is partially due to the secrecy of practice, the unwritten and undocumented historical development, and the conflicting oral history accounts of its beginnings.

What can be said is that karate is an Okinawan martial art that was heavily influenced by the fighting arts in China. These Chinese arts have in their roots gong fu (kung fu) or quanfa (fist way).

The major style of gong fu has also been referred to as Shaolin, known for its quick snapping and thrusting techniques. The Shaolin style was created by Bodhidarma (Ta-mo, Lao-tsu). Dharma was said to have been invited by the Chinese Emperor Wu to teach Buddhist Law at the Shaolin monastery in China's Hunan province (approximately 520 AD).[3]

Bodhidarma (founder of the Zen sect of Buddhism) was supposedly born in India. Legend says that he traveled on foot from India to China. Once there, he developed the Ekiken and Senzui sutras and taught the monks accordingly.[4] Ekiken refers to the disciplining and strengthening the body, while Senzui refers to strengthening the will and polishing the mind.[5] Together, they formed the basis for the Chinese fist hand or gong fu.

Gong-fu or quanfa is documented in the *Bubishi* (the bible of karate). The *Bubishi* represents the original precepts of self-defense by the ancient masters in China. There are actually two *Bubishi*. One is a voluminous text on the art of war with 240 chapters that deal with strategic warfare of a nation (naval, strategy, troop deployment, occupation, etc.). The other *Bubishi* is the one that is discussed in this chapter. This *Bubishi* contains thirty-two articles and is said to be the original documentation of Chinese gong fu.[6]

The ideogram for the word *Bubishi* when broken down means the following: bu = military, bi = to provide or prepare, and shi = record. So when we put them together it means a manual of military preparation. The manual itself instructs on the offensive and defensive techniques of civil fighting traditions and also instructs and promotes the more subtle understanding of uncovering the true self and polishing the human spirit (revealing the broad understanding of the martial art). In other words, martial arts become the conduit for the deeper understanding of the self.[7]

The author and time period of this document are unknown, but it appears to have surfaced in the southern Chinese province of Fujian and more specifically in and around the city of Fuzhou in the late 17th or early 18th century.[8]

Okinawa became a tributary of China in the latter part of the 14th century. Basically they were a province of China. This meant that there were representatives from China who were sent to Okinawa as political and military ambassadors. The Okinawans also visited the Chinese mainland mainly in the city of Fuzhou in the Fujian province of southern China.

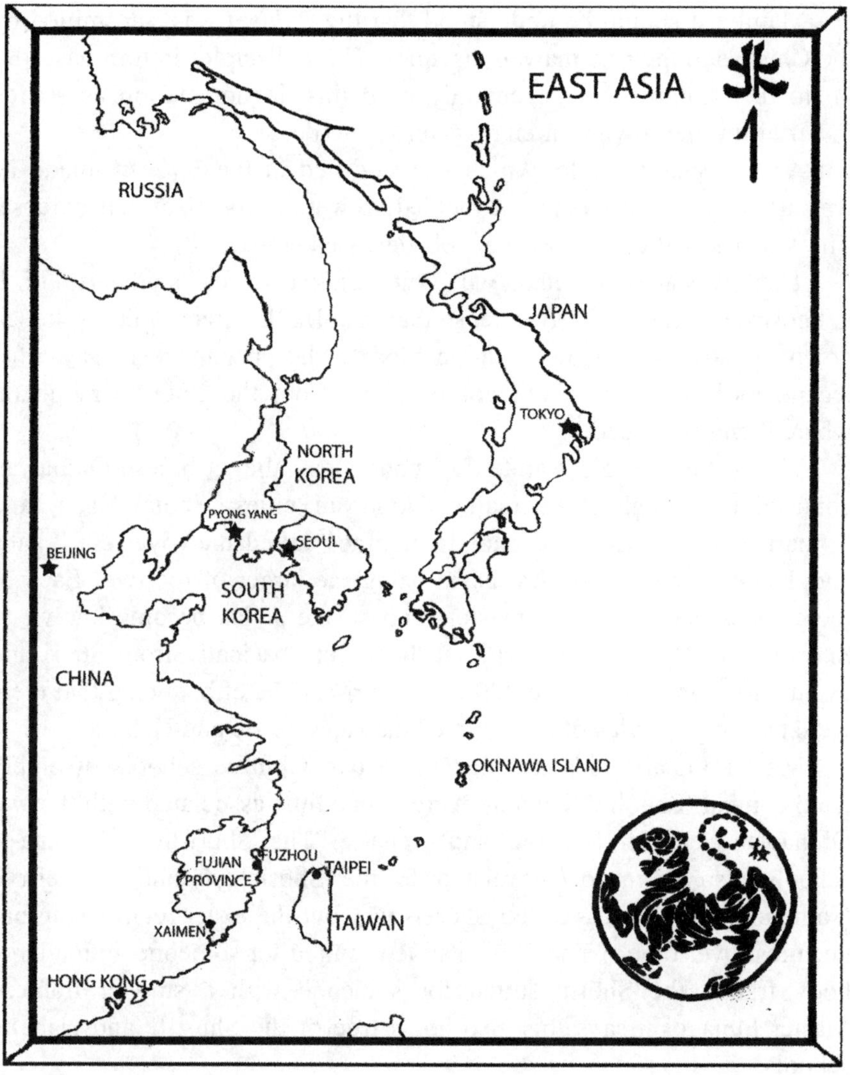

This relationship between the two countries is an important part of the puzzle in helping to understand the transmission of the *Bubishi* from China to Okinawa. It is presumed that this *Bubishi* made its way from Fuzhou to Okinawa sometime during the mid-to late 19th century, but exactly how remains speculative.

Mainly, it should be understood that the *Bubishi* was transmitted by the Chinese to their Okinawan disciples. These disciples in turn passed it on to their juniors who eventually used this documentation as source material for their own written texts on karate-dō.

As the Shaolin style, which was codified in the *Bubishi*, made its way to the Ryūkyū Islands, it melded with local forms of self-defense. The Japanese called this form of self-defense kempo.

There was also the Shang wu (Wutang), known for its powerful ki. It is known as a form of self-defense that enables the practitioner to knock down an adversary with a single blow.[9] Master Funakoshi says that legend indicates this school got its name from the Chinese mountain where it was practiced.[10]

The lineage of karate-dō continues the Chinese-Okinawan connection through three major Okinawan cities: Shuri, Naha, and Tomari.[11] Shuri was the capital, sometimes called the royal city. Naha and Tomari were port cities, Naha being the larger of the two. Each of these cities had their own masters and so the styles became known as Shuri-te and Naha-te. Tomari's teachers were basically from Shuri and eventually Tomari-te converged with Shuri-te. The effect being that there were two major styles of karate in Okinawa, Shuri-te and Naha-te.[12]

Master Funakoshi states that these two Chinese schools of empty hand combat (Shaolin, Wutang) were at one time associated with the two Okinawan schools, Shuri-te and Naha-te. The Shuri-te and Naha-te schools also seem to be related to the Shōrin-ryū and Shōkei-ryū (sometimes incorrectly called Shōrei-ryū), but the exact relationship has been lost over time.[13] The Shōkei style is suited for someone with a large body frame, the Shōrin suited for someone with a smaller frame.[14] Master Funakoshi says this also holds true of the Shuri-te and Naha-te schools.

The systemization of this Okinawan martial art known as te or bushi-no-te can be seen through the appearance of the *Bubishi* in Okinawa and the spread of instruction by the original masters and experts of the art. At this time the empty-handed form of self-defense, which began as an Okinawan martial art, had come into contact with the different styles of Chinese gong fu to produce a new and dynamic martial art (karate).

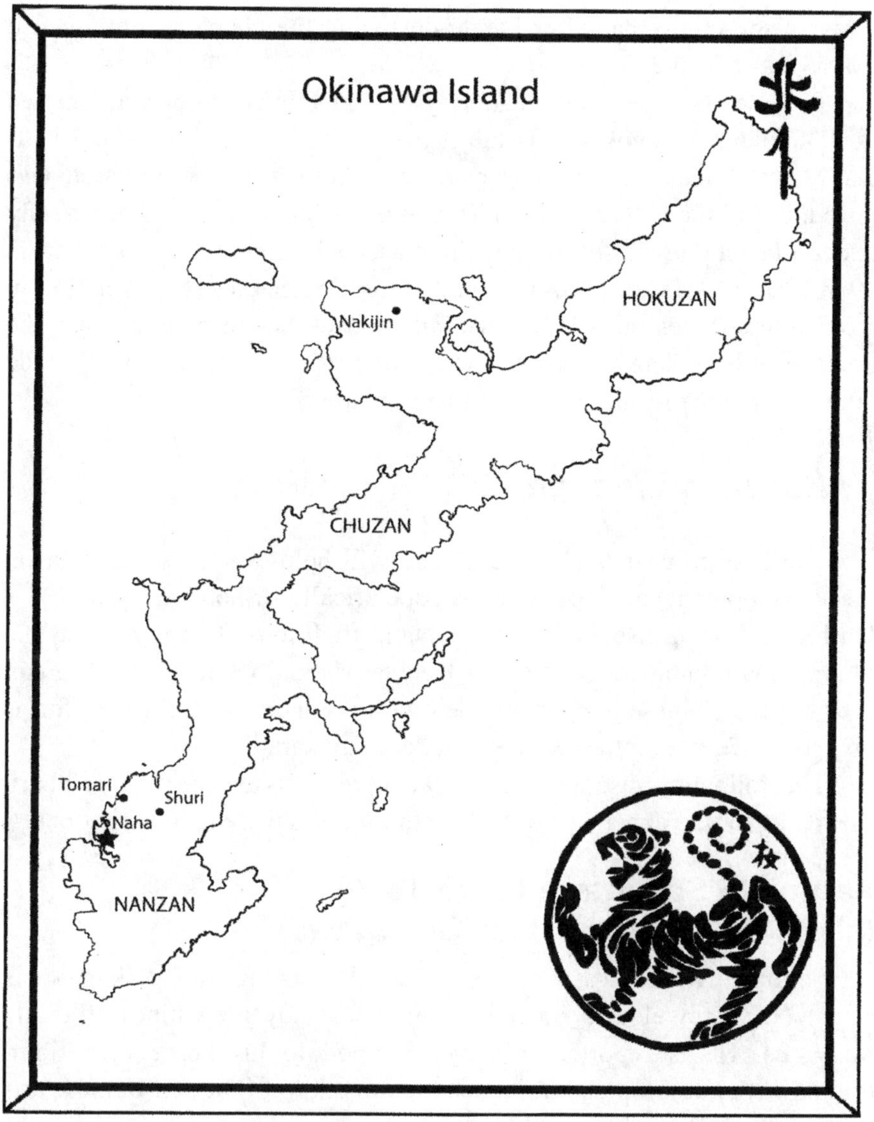

The lineage of karate progressed into the "Japanization" of karate by Master Gichin Funakoshi. Under Master Funakoshi, this Okinawan method of self-defense, which had been called "Chinese-hand" (using the character pronounced "kara" that meant Chinese) developed into the "way of the empty hand" or karate-dō (using the character pronounced "kara" that meant empty).

The school of practice created by Master Funakoshi became known as "Shotokan." Shotokan was the name of the first dōjō (training hall) that Master Funakoshi built in Japan. This Shotokan school of karate was introduced to the U.S. by Master Tsutomu Ohshima, who studied directly under Master Funakoshi at Japan's Waseda University in Tokyo from 1948 to 1953. Master Ohshima created the first Shotokan association in the United States in 1955. Ohshima Sensei has further refined the practice of Shotokan Karate, and today thousands of students worldwide practice Shotokan Karate — Ohshima in many countries.

Karate's Lineage

The lineage chart on the next page will help to shed some light on the development of karate, more specifically, Shotokan Karate — Ohshima. I have also included the Naha traditions (Goju-ryū) and the Shuri/Naha combined tradition of Kenwa Mabuni (Shito Ryū). We can see how the Chinese gong fu melded with the indigenous fighting forms Okinawan Te to eventually create modern day karate.

The following discussion looks at the experts on the lineage chart. The dates for the experts prior to Gichin Funakoshi are approximations.

Satunishi Sakugawa (1733-1815) (also known as "Karate" Sakugawa)

Satunishi Sakugawa, who was referred to as "Karate" Sakugawa is said to have traveled to Fuzhou (China) to study the Chinese fighting traditions. He is reported to have returned to his home near Shuri (Okinawa) to develop and influence the directions of the self-defense arts there. Sakugawa had incredible physical prowess, and was employed as the head of security for a prominent commercial shipping firm.[15]

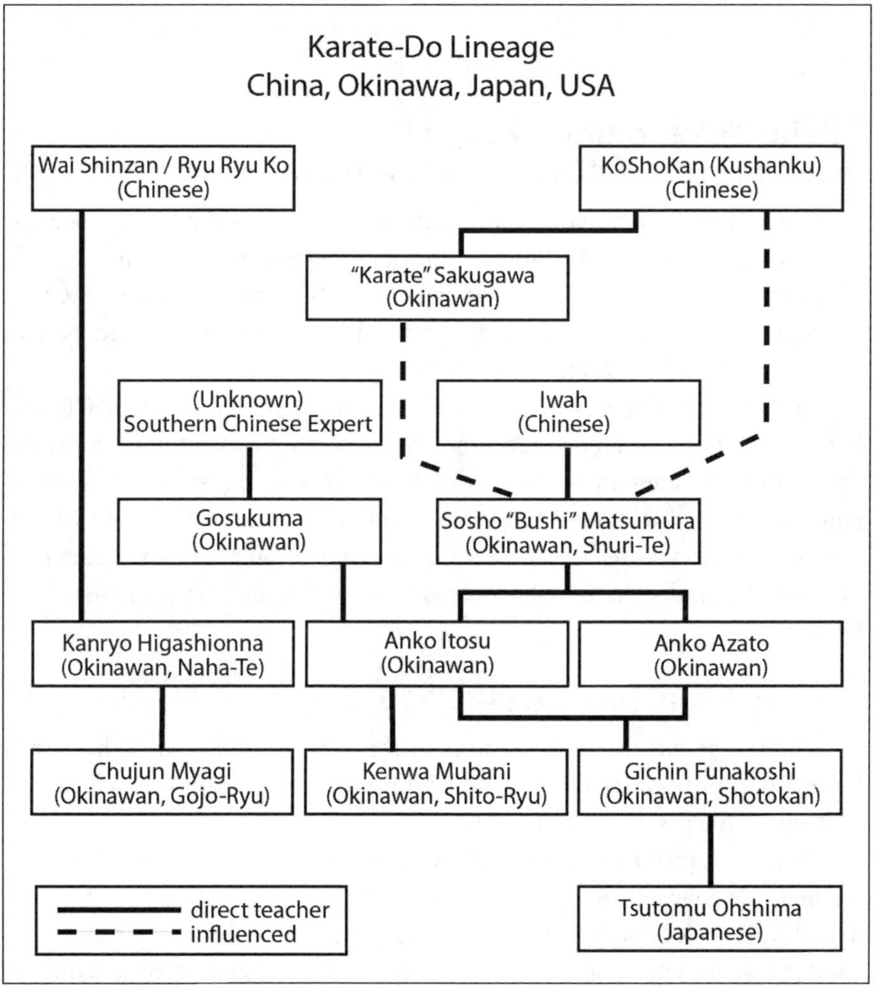

Figure 3: Karate-dō lineage from China to Shotokan — Ohshima.

KoShoKun (Kushanku) (1700s)

KoShoKun was a Chinese cultural attaché who came to Okinawa with several personal disciples. He was said to be an expert in kempo (Chinese boxing). He taught and developed the Chinese hand in Okinawa from the mid-1750s to the early 1760s. Legend and oral tradition maintain he was a teacher of Karate Sakugawa.[16] He is credited with introducing the kata known as Kwanku. Tradition also says he introduced the hikite (pulling hand).

Soshu Matsumura (1796-1893) (also known as "Bushi" Matsumura)

Soshu Matsumura, sometimes known as "Bushi" Matsumura became a major influence in developing the karate movement in and around Shuri (Okinawa). Matsumura studied in the Fujian province of China (studying under gong fu master Iwah) and also under the direction of Okinawan Master "Karate" Sakugawa.

Under Matsumura's direction the fighting arts tradition of Chinese hand and Okinawan hand became synthesized to eventually form the style Shuri-te (later to be known as Shōrin-Ryu). Matsumura served as chief bodyguard to three Okinawan kings. (For a period of time Master Anko Itosu served as his understudy.)[17] Matsumura is also credited as one of the individuals who introduced the kata Passai (Bassai) to Okinawa.

Kanryo Higashionna (1853-1915)

Kanryo Higashionna was born in the Okinawa city of Naha. He is known as the founder of Naha-te (the precursor to Goju-ryu which was created by his disciple Chojun Miyagi).

Master Kanryo traveled to the Chinese city of Fuzhou in 1868 as a student. He learned the gong fu martial arts from Masters Wai Shinzan and Ryu Ryu-Ko, both Shaolin Temple experts. He returned from China fourteen years later and developed Naha-te, which instructed not only in ways of combat but also in the spiritual, moral, and ethical aspects of a martial art.[18]

Anko Azato (1827-1906)

Both Azato and Anko Itosu were the direct teachers of Gichin Funakoshi. Gichin Funakoshi states that Master Azato was "unsurpassed in all Okinawa in the art of Karate."[19] Azato was an aristocrat who owned his own castle. He was lord of Azato village located between

Naha and Shuri, was a high-ranking military officer and very close to the king as the king's privy councilor.

Funakoshi became Azato's only disciple and actually received his first training from Azato. "Azato was tall and broad-shouldered and had fiery, piercing eyes, very ready calling to mind the Bushi of old."[20] Azato was also said to be an expert in kendo, archery, and horsemanship.

Anko Itosu (1832-1915)

Itosu and Azato had the same first name. These two masters were the direct disciples of "Bushi" Matsumura. Itosu's appearance was the complete opposite of Azato's. He was of normal height with a muscular chest. He had a beard and was said to have the look of a gentle child. Itosu had tremendous strength and a powerful grip. It was reported that he could crush a shoot of bamboo with his bare hands.[21] Itosu also worked in the royal court with Azato. Supposedly Azato recommended his friend Itosu to serve as the king's private secretary.[22] Itosu is credited with creating the Pinan (Heian) Katas drawing from the more advanced Shotokan forms Kwanku and Bassai.[23] Itosu introduced karate training to the public school systems in Okinawa at the beginning of the 20th century. Both Itosu and Azato served as direct teachers of Gichin Funakoshi.

Gichin Funakoshi (1868-1957)

Gichin Funakoshi was born in Shuri province in Okinawa in 1868. Funakoshi learned from the two great masters, Azato and Itosu. He also studied under "Bushi" Matsumura and Kiyuna, Tōonno (of Naha), and Niigaki (who was a renowned Confucian scholar).[24]

Master Funakoshi is often given the title of "Father of Modern Karate." With the leading karate men of the time, he began to publicly introduce karate in Okinawa (circa 1906).[25] Funakoshi was further privileged to travel, in 1916, to the Japanese Butoku-den in Kyoto (the official center of Japanese martial arts) to demonstrate karate.[26]

He publicly introduced karate to Japan in 1922 at the First National Athletic Exhibition in Tokyo. This was done at the request of the Department of Education of Okinawa Prefecture.[27] (Master Funakoshi was a schoolteacher.) It was at this public demonstration that Gichin Funakoshi was invited by the famous judo master Kanō Jigorō to teach at the Kodokan.[28] Jigorō himself requested lessons. Master Funakoshi began to demonstrate and teach the art of karate to many groups in and around Tokyo.

Master Funakoshi also published the first book (1922) on the subject of karate, *Ryukyu Kempo: Karate*. The Master wrote two more versions of this book, *Karate-Dō Kyōhan* (first edition and second edition). The second edition was not completed by Master Funakoshi because he died prior to its completion. The first edition of *Karate-Dō Kyōhan* was translated into English by Tsutomu Ohshima in 1973.

Master Funakoshi is called the Father of Modern Karate because he was instrumental not only in publicly introducing karate to Japan but also in developing this method of self-defense into a martial art (similar to judō and kendō). That change began with the changing of the original ideogram for karate (which meant Chinese hand) to the new character for karate which meant empty or void. (The ideogram can also be pronounced "ku.") This kara (empty) represented spiritual emancipation and the inner void (world within).[29] So karate with this ideogram meant not only that one physically had no weapons, but also that one embraced the metaphysical. In other words, one also practiced this martial art in pursuit of inner discovery.

The Dō was added to the ending in the same manner as other Japanese martial arts (kendō, judō, budō). This dō means way or path. Karate-jutsu therefore became karate-dō and soon, through the efforts of Master Funakoshi, the original Te or Chinese Te grew into an officially recognized martial art in Japanese society.

This was the beginnings of the "Japanization" of Okinawan self-defense into a bona fide way of polishing the human spirit.

Funakoshi's style of practicing karate became known as Shotokan Karate. Shoto was the Master's pen name meaning "pine waves," Kan means "house" or the place where Shoto's karate is practiced.[30] Shotokan Karate was introduced to the United States by Tsutomu Ohshima.

Shotokan Tiger

Gichin Funakoshi's pen name "Shoto" literally means "pine waves," and today is synonymous with the tiger symbol and Shotokan Karate-dō. But few people understand the relationship of Shoto to what is commonly known as the "Shotokan Tiger."

When Gichin Funakoshi was a young man, he enjoyed walking in solitude among the pine trees which surrounded his home town of Shuri. After a hard day of teaching in the local school and several more hours of strenuous karate practice, he would often walk up Mount Torao and meditate among the pine trees. Mount Torao is a very narrow, heavily wooded mountain which, when viewed from a distance, resembles a tiger's tail. The name "Torao" in fact literally means "tiger's tail."

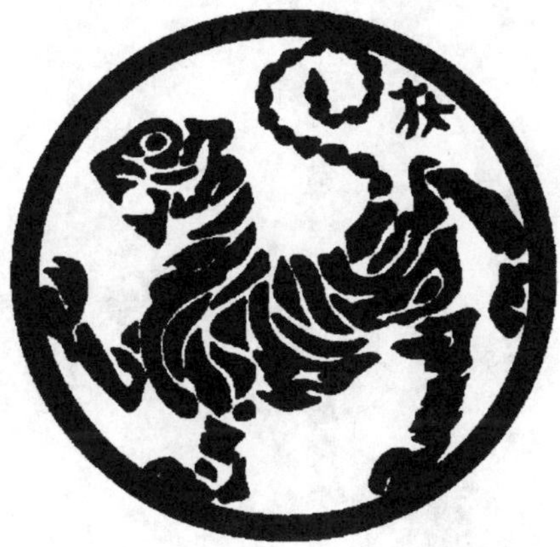

In later life, Funakoshi explained that the cool breezes which blew among the pines made the trees whisper like waves breaking on the shore. Thus, since he gained his greatest poetic inspirations while walking there, he chose the pen name of Shoto, "pine waves."

The tiger which is commonly used as the symbol for Shotokan Karate is a traditional Chinese design which implies that "the tiger never sleeps." Symbolized in the Shotokan tiger, therefore, is the keen alertness of the wakeful tiger and the serenity of the peaceful mind which Gichin Funakoshi experienced while listening to the pine waves on Tiger's Tail Mountain.

Tsutomu Ohshima (1930)

Tsutomu Ohshima was born on August 6, 1930. Ohshima Sensei began his martial arts training at age five in sumo wrestling. He continued with this until he was fifteen. He also studied kendo from eight to fifteen and judo from nine to thirteen.

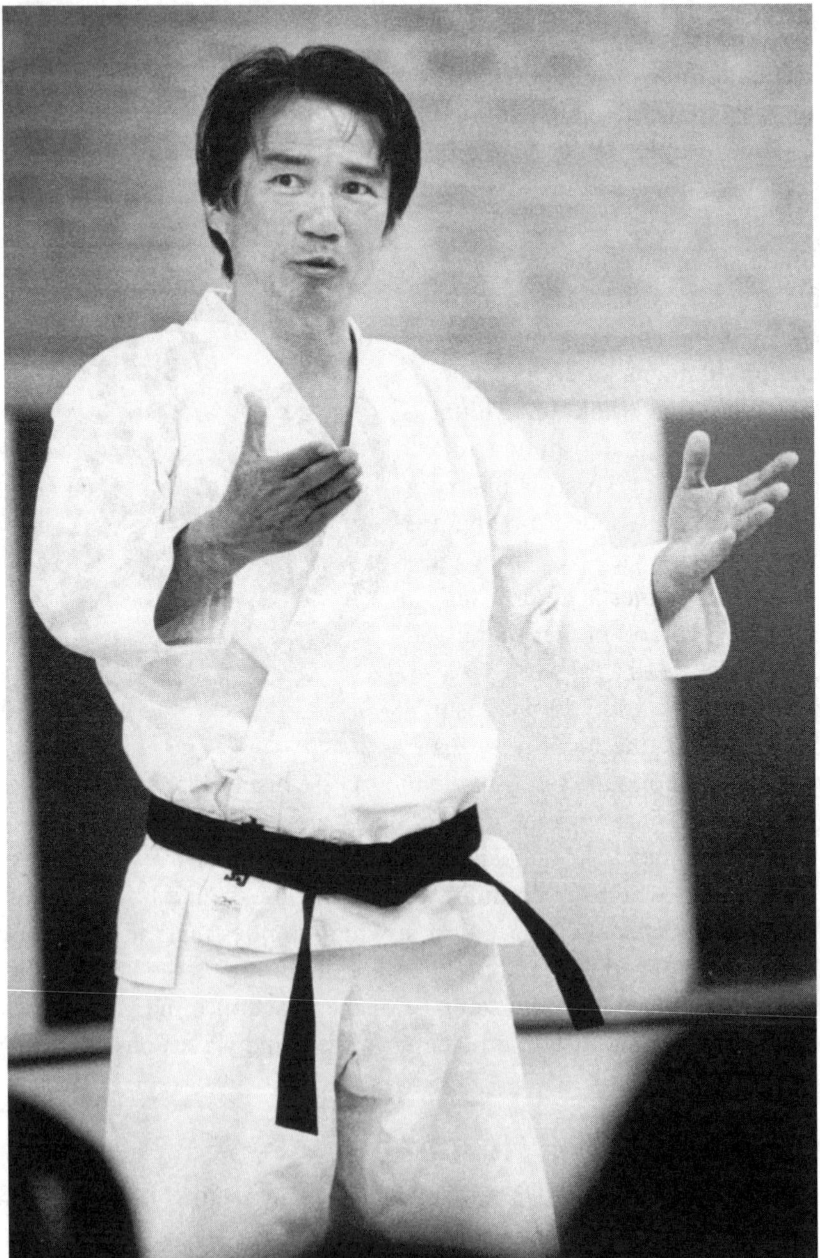

Photograph reprinted with the permission of Ohshima Sensei and Shotokan Karate of America.

Ohshima Sensei was the direct pupil of Gichin Funakoshi at Waseda University (Tokyo) from 1948 to 1953. He served as the captain of the Waseda Karate Club. Ohshima Sensei also trained with his seniors Hiroshi Noguchi, Shigeru Egami, and Toshio Kamata-Wantanabe.[31]

Ohshima Sensei came to the United States to do graduate studies at the University of Southern California in 1955. In 1956 Ohshima Sensei introduced Shotokan Karate to the United States. A year later he formed the first college karate club at the California Institute of Technology. In 1959 he formed the Southern California Karate Association, which ten years later became Shotokan Karate of America. Today, there are no less than 15 different countries with affiliate karate organizations.[32]

Ohshima Sensei started the traditional practice of Special Trainings in the United States. These trainings are three- or four-day events which challenge the participants to push themselves beyond their perceived physical and mental limitations. This is a very important element in the traditional karate practitioners' development in karate-dō.

Ohshima Sensei was also given permission by Master Funakoshi's family to translate *Karate-Dō Kyōhan: The Master Text*, which was published in 1973, into English. *Karate-Dō Kyōhan* is the official reference for Shotokan Karate — Ohshima. For any questions about techniques in this book or in class, please refer to *Karate-Dō Kyōhan.* Ohshima Sensei has continued to refine the practice of Shotokan Karate through his own practice and through study with his respected seniors, Hiroshi Noguchi, Shigeru Egami, Toshio Kamata-Wantanabe, Tadao Okuyama, and Matsuo Shibuya. Those who train and have practiced (Ohshima Method) with Ohshima Sensei refer to this method as Shotokan Karate — Ohshima. Today, Ohshima Sensei resides in Santa Barbara, California, and continues to instruct students from around the world.

Summary

We can see that the indigenous forms of Okinawan self defense, te (hand) or bushi-no-te (warriors' hand), became influenced by the Chinese gong fu and the Chinese martial arts experts. We can also see how the *Bubishi* could have been transmitted from China to Okinawa, possibly by one or more of the experts, "Karate" Sakugawa, KoShoKun, "Bushi" Matsumura, Kanryo Higashionna, or Anko Itosu.

These experts, with the Chinese experts who visited their tributary Okinawa, were all possible transmitters of this document. This document was very instrumental in helping to develop karate into a "Way" or martial art. However, just as important were the experts who personally transmitted this art from senior to junior.

Suggested Reading

Karate-Dō Kyōhan by Gichin Funakoshi, translated by Tsutomu Ohshima. Chapter 1. Introduction.

---

[1] Gichin Funakoshi, *Karate Jutsu*, p. 25.
[2] Gichin Funakoshi, *Karate-Dō: My Way of Life*, p. 29.
[3] Gichin Funakoshi, *Karate-Dō Nyūmon*, p. 20.
[4] *Ibid.*, pp. 20-21.
[5] *Ibid.*
[6] Patrick McCarthy, *The Bible of Karate: Bubishi*, pp. 26-27.
[7] *Ibid.*, p. 23.
[8] *Ibid.*, p. 30.
[9] Gichin Funakoshi, *Karate-Dō Nyūmon*, p. 20.
[10] Gichin Funakoshi, *Karate-Dō: My Way of Life*, p. 37.
[11] Lawrence Kane, Kris Wilder, *The Way of Kata*, p. 4.
[12] *Ibid.*
[13] Gichin Funakoshi, *Karate-Dō: My Way of Life*, p. 38.
[14] *Ibid.*
[15] Patrick McCarthy, *The Bible of Karate: Bubishi*, p. 34.
[16] *Ibid.*, pp. 33-34
[17] *Ibid.*, p. 51.
[18] *Ibid.*, pp. 34, 39.
[19] Gichin Funakoshi, *Karate-Dō: My Way of Life*, p. 3.
[20] Gichin Funakoshi, *Karate-Dō: Nyūmon*, p. 33.
[21] Gichin Funakoshi, *Karate-Dō: My Way of Life*, pp. 16-19.
[22] Gichin Funakoshi, *Karate-Dō: Nyūmon*, p. 30.
[23] Tsutomu Ohshima, *Notes on Training*, p. 11.
[24] Gichin Funakoshi, *Karate-Dō: My Way of Life*, p. 13.
[25] Gichin Funakoshi, *Karate-Dō Kyōhan*, pp. 9-10.
[26] Gichin Funakoshi, *Karate-Dō Kyōhan*, p. 10.
[27] Gichin Funakoshi, *Karate-Dō Kyōhan*, p. 10.
[28] Gichin Funakoshi, *Karate-Dō: My Way of Life*, pp. 69-70.
[29] Gichin Funakoshi, *Karate-Dō: My Way of Life*, pp. 34-36.
[30] Gichin Funakoshi, *Karate-Dō: My Way of Life*, pp. 83-86.
[31] Shotokan Karate of America. SKA.org.
[32] *Ibid.*

2. Preparing to Practice

One of the greatest parts of Martial Arts is that at the same time we are polishing our physical movements, we are also polishing our minds and thus becoming better persons.[1]

Tsutomu Ohshima
Shihan, Shotokan Karate of America

Mentality and Conduct

There is a certain amount of formalism that is maintained in traditional karate or martial arts practice. To understand martial arts, a student needs to understand the formality that surrounds it.

Bow (Rei)

An important aspect of the formalism in martial arts is found in the bow or rei. Performing the bow well shows your respect for your opponent, for your teacher, for your dōjō, and for life itself. All of our gestures in life are very important, especially rei because this simple act sets the tone, helping you to develop correct behavior. Rei displays the human attributes of dignity and respect, with the eventual outcome of having these qualities become part of our normal behavior.[2] Our practice of karate-dō must always begin and end with rei.

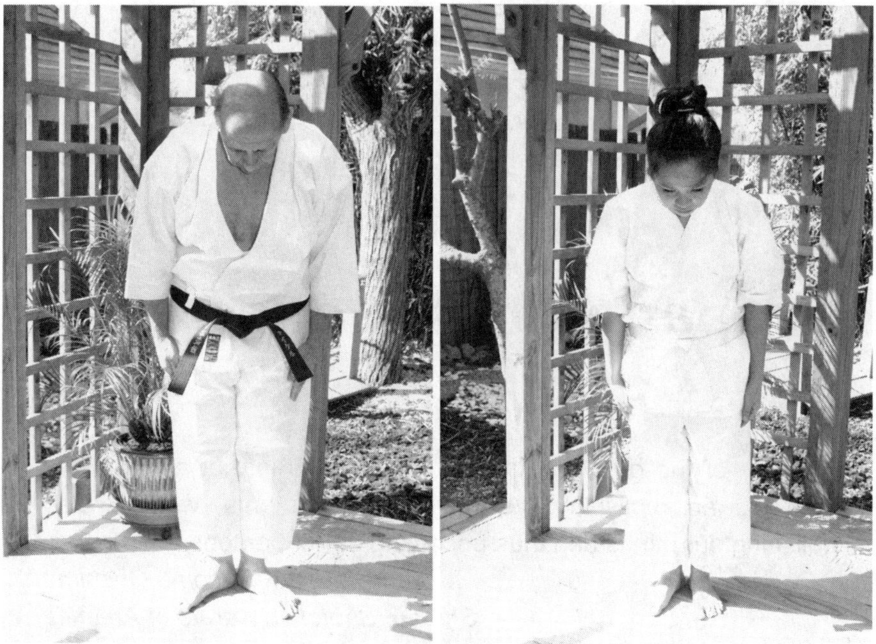

Figure 4: Rei.

Some may scoff at this, or even argue that you can't learn to defend yourself by being respectful and showing patience and self-discipline. This instruction, however, is in karate-dō or the Way of the Empty Hand, signifying that the student is seeking to polish who he or she is by practicing and perfecting both the physical and mental skills of karate. Karate-dō is more than just punching or kicking. In essence, it is an avenue for becoming a more productive and mature human being who will contribute in a positive way to society.

The "dō" of karate-dō, kendō, aikidō, judō, or kyūdō signifies a method of teaching that particular art that enables a person to unravel the secret nature of their own mind through dedicated practice and to discover the true self. It strips away our small, self-centered ego. It develops in each of us, who continue to practice, the ability to discover our own true nature.[3] (Refer to chapter 1 on the changing of kara (Chinese) to kara (empty, void).

Dress and Demeanor

Beginning students may or may not need to worry about specific clothing or outfits. Ask your instructor for the requirements for your particular class. The usual situation is that you may wear a gi (training uniform) if you have one, but loose, comfortable clothing such as sweatpants and T-shirts may also be worn by beginners.

Students will practice with bare feet. No hats will be allowed in class. Head sweatbands are permitted. The hair should be secured and not be able to fall into your eyes and face. Jewelry should be kept to a minimum. This is done mainly for safety, but also for a neat and clean appearance.

Attendance and Behavior

To obtain the maximum benefit of the class, regular attendance is not just required. It is a necessity if a student wants to build any real foundation. This is especially true for the first several months when the student will be introduced to many important new techniques as well as the theoretical concepts, discussions, and demonstrations that help form the core formational values.

Active participation is extremely important. I mentioned before that we are complex beings: intellectual, emotional, physical, and spiritual. This means that physically showing-up for class is not enough. We must give the class our full attention intellectually and emotionally, too.

Your observation of the demonstrated techniques by the instructor and your ability to imitate and practice them in repetitive fashion will help your body to understand unconsciously (through muscle memory) the correct muscles that need to be employed. The body and mind will then function as an automatic response when the technique is executed. At this stage, please be open to your instructor's correction of your movements, for it is extremely important to have proper form.

No gum chewing or food will be allowed once class has begun. Cross or belligerent behavior during class will not be tolerated. Students are not permitted to initiate challenges or be engaged in any form of dueling. Students who do this will be removed from class.

Mysterious Oriental Art

The heading is listed as "Mysterious Oriental Art." Sometimes karate-dō or Eastern martial arts are considered mysterious and esoteric. Actually, the heading should read "Mysterious Oriental Art That Isn't Mysterious."

Our introduction to the practice of karate-dō should begin with our understanding of self-defense. Hopefully, we can move forward and grow in this understanding. When trying to reach the pinnacle of a mountain, there are many different paths. As one arrives at the base of the last approach to the summit, he will discover that all of the paths have converged to a central point.[4] That being said, the real meaning for the word budō (the way of combat) is to stop combat. There is also a deeper underlying meaning here, and that is to actually stop the abuse of power.

Studying karate-dō means that we practice to prevent the mentality of abusiveness. Many times, our initial reaction to ending a confrontation is to use some type of force. As we begin to train, we must strive to rethink our actions when confronted with these situations.

Often our behavior itself invites negative, destructive, or harmful situations. Retired Lt. Col. David Grossman states our chances of being molested can be greatly reduced simply by not looking or acting like a victim. Lt. Col. Grossman teaches a psychology and military science course at the United States Military Academy at West Point. Grossman, a former army ranger, has combined his experiences to study the root causes of violent crimes and the process of healing the victims of violence in war and peace.[5]

Professor Grossman conducted a research program on convicts who were convicted of violent predatory crimes on other human beings. His research indicated that the criminals preyed on their victims similarly to how large predatory cats stalk their prey. Both picked out the weakest to attack.[6]

These criminals related that they singled out individuals by body language: slumped walk, passive behavior, and a lack of awareness. Professor Grossman states, "However, when potential victims gave cues that indicated they would not go easily, the cons said they would walk away. If the criminals sensed the target was a counter-predator, that is a sheepdog, they would leave them alone unless there was no other choice but to engage."[7]

I thought it was very interesting how Professor Grossman divided people in his study into three major categories: sheep, wolves, and sheepdogs. His feeling is that most of society (sheep) is happy and productive with neither the capacity for violence nor do they prepare for any type of dangerous or confrontational situation.

Wolves are just the opposite. They prey on the innocent and weak of our society, on the sheep. Sheepdogs, however, understand about the wolves of our society and are willing and able to confront them when necessary (even a physical confrontation). But there is a big difference between wolves and sheepdogs. The difference is the moral and ethical conduct of the sheepdogs (many of these individuals are drawn to the military or law enforcement; some are also drawn to traditional martial arts training). Grossman continues by stating that sheepdogs never use force for personal gain but only for the protection of self or others and for preserving the common good.[8] Engaging in a physical or violent confrontation however is not something that the martial artist should take lightly or with a cavalier attitude.

If in the course of our lives a confrontation is unavoidable, then we must use our karate training to the best of our ability and not shrink from the situation we find ourselves embroiled in. We must strike swiftly and with the intent of ending the confrontation quickly.

We are truly called as practitioners to stop the conflict. As we grow in our understanding of karate-dō, we continuously build our martial arts structure. The closer we come to the pinnacle of understanding, the more we begin to comprehend the ideogram for bu in the word budō, which means to stop the combat.

Beginning the Traditional Work-out

Meditation (Mokusō)

Mokusō (pronounced moh-kso) is literally translated as meditation. It is done at the beginning and at the end of each practice session. This is a short period when we clear our minds of the baggage that we all carry with us. We do this in order that we might be able to better focus on the upcoming training session.

This is similar to the concept of mushin (in Zen) where we clear or empty our minds. In kumite (combat), this is known as mushin no shin (mind of no mind), that is, not being attached to any thought, concept, or feeling. To make this beginning meditation, we kneel in what is called *seiza*. For men the form is usually done with the knees slightly apart. For women the knees are usually together.

There is no great secret to making mokusō. One should always kneel keeping the back as straight as possible, and not drooping your shoulders. Your nose and naval area should be almost vertically connected. The palms of the hand will be on your thighs either up (open) or down with the thumb and index finger coming slightly together.

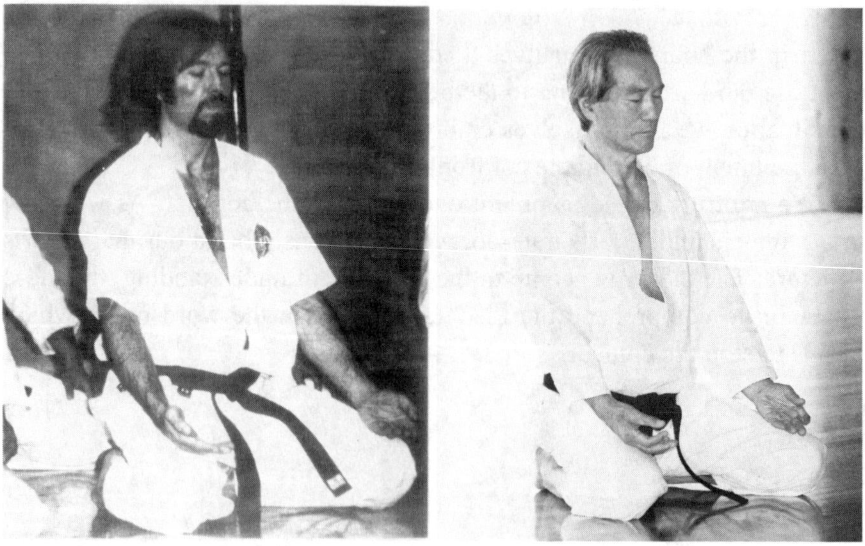

Figure 5: Don DePree and Ohshima Sensei in mokusō.

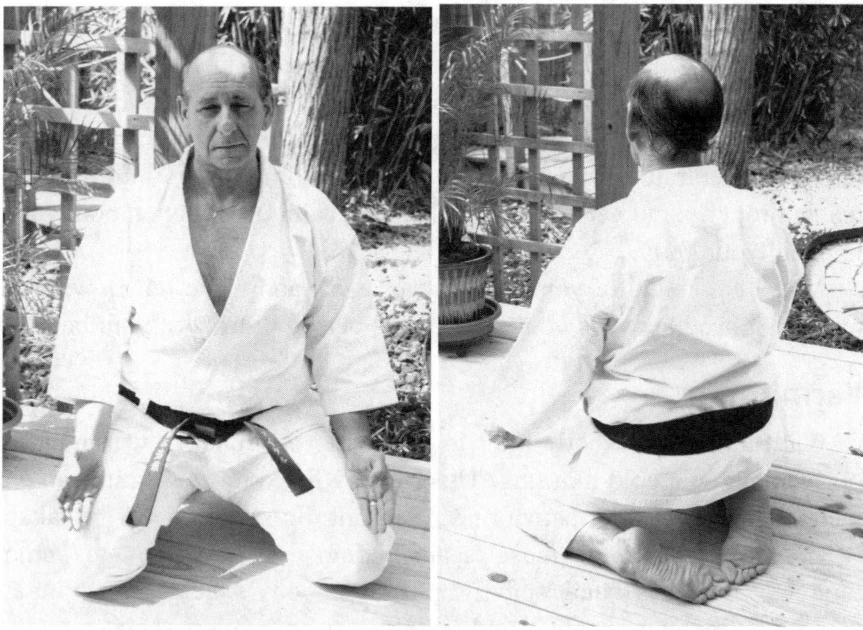

Figure 6: Mokusō posture for males.

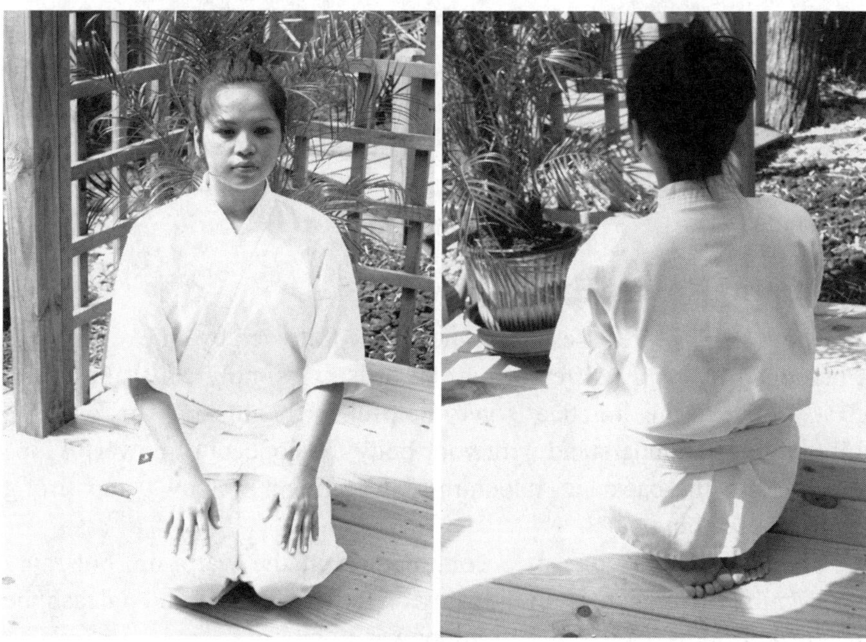

Figure 7: Mokusō posture for females.

Next at the command mokusō, close your eyes lightly and begin to concentrate on your breathing, especially in your lower abdomen or tanden area. The tongue is placed behind your upper teeth. Breathe in and out quietly, inhaling through your nose and exhaling through your mouth. Concentrate on your tanden (lower abdomen). Learning how to breathe properly and very deeply will have a calming effect on both your mind and your body.

At the command of yame, open your eyes, and make rei. Bow from your waist, head between your open palms placed in front of your body.

Warming up

Warming up your body prior to practicing is similar to warming up your vehicle on a cold morning. This activity helps to transition from an inactive state to a more active one. Warming up should never be taken for granted. It helps the muscles and cardiovascular system to pump blood to your heart and slightly raise the body's core temperature. Hopefully, this can be done with a minimal amount of shock to your body systems.

Warming up is just what it says. It's to warm-up. It is not a time for intense stretching. It is simply done to loosen and warm your muscles. Combined with mokusō, warming up also mentally prepares you for more intense physical activity. Warming up should always precede your actual class and should be done with moderation without extreme jumps or stretches.

Push and Resist Exercise

The warm-up exercises are immediately followed by an exercise that is practiced by many different martial artists. I simply call it push and resist. I believe this practice is very helpful for beginners. This exercise will help you to understand with your body the concept of powerful hips connected to the back leg, underarms, little fingers, elbows, and strong powerful breathing.

This exercise is done as a continuation of the warm-up, but more specifically, it begins to train the body on how to harness and unleash the center of our power-base, the strong powerful hips.

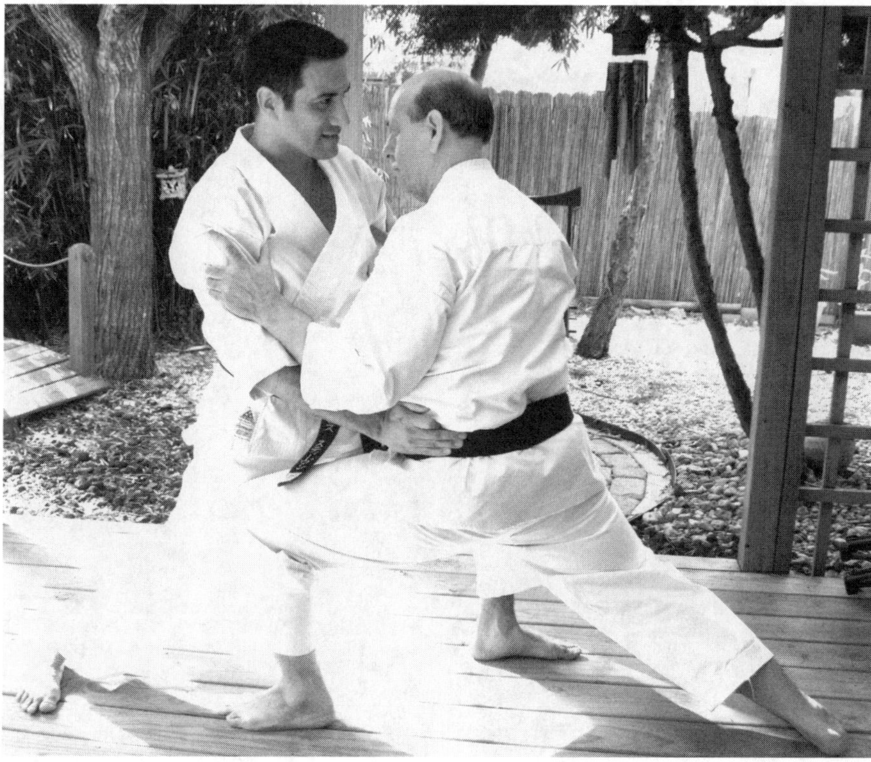

Figure 8: Push and resist practice.

Suggested Reading

Karate-Dō Kyōhan by Gichin Funakoshi, translated by Tsutomu Ohshima. Chapter 1. Introduction.

---

[1] Tsutomu Ohshima, *Notes on Training*, p. 2.
[2] Taisen Deshimaru, *The Zen Way to The Martial Arts*, pp. 88-89.
[3] *Ibid.*, p. 11.
[4] Kane, Wilder, *The Way of Kata*, p. 37.
[5] *Ibid.*, pp. 153-154
[6] *Ibid.*
[7] *Ibid.*
[8] *Ibid.*

3. Foundational Structure: Core Values

Patience determines the depth of perfection of all aspects of oneself, so be patient, and give plenty of time to all aspects of karate practice. (Instead of learning 1,000 different techniques, learn 1,000 things about one technique. Then when you learn how to make one technique truly effective, that understanding, will carry through to all techniques.)[1]

Don DePree, Shotokan Karate of America

Hips, stances with their power lines and pulling hand, breathing, and eyes are the foundation we build our karate techniques on. In this chapter we will look at these foundational concepts.

Hips

Ohshima Sensei says, "The center of human strength is the hips, all other movements have to go with the motion of the hips. Someone who moves his hips idealistically we call a strong man, an expert."[2]

The hips serve as the center that generates the power in the various movements of karate-dō. You will soon realize, however, that moving the hips in any direction is not only hard work, but is paramount in developing the necessary fundamental understanding of practice. The hips basically move in three different ways: straight-line from back to front or from front to back), straight line from side to side, and rotating or turning.[3]

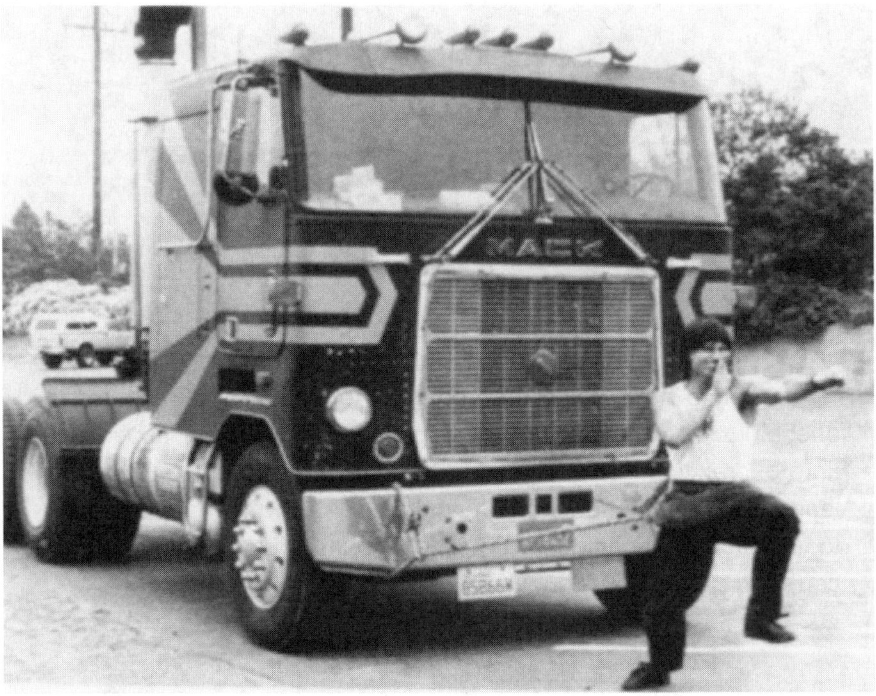

Figure 9: Tom Muzila practices making powerful hips.

Power Lines

Correct form in any technique can unleash the powerful untapped strength and energy of a human being. Examples of this form are easily demonstrated by using a simple zenkutsu-dachi (front stance) form with the arms placed properly for penetration with an oi-zuki (front punch) and gyaku-zuki (reverse-punch). Please refer to the examples of these concepts by studying the following illustrations.

Notice that when the body alignment is incorrect the power generated by the body (mainly through the hips) cannot be transferred.

You should take note of the proper body alignment, and how it realistically connects to a successful and penetrating technique.[4]

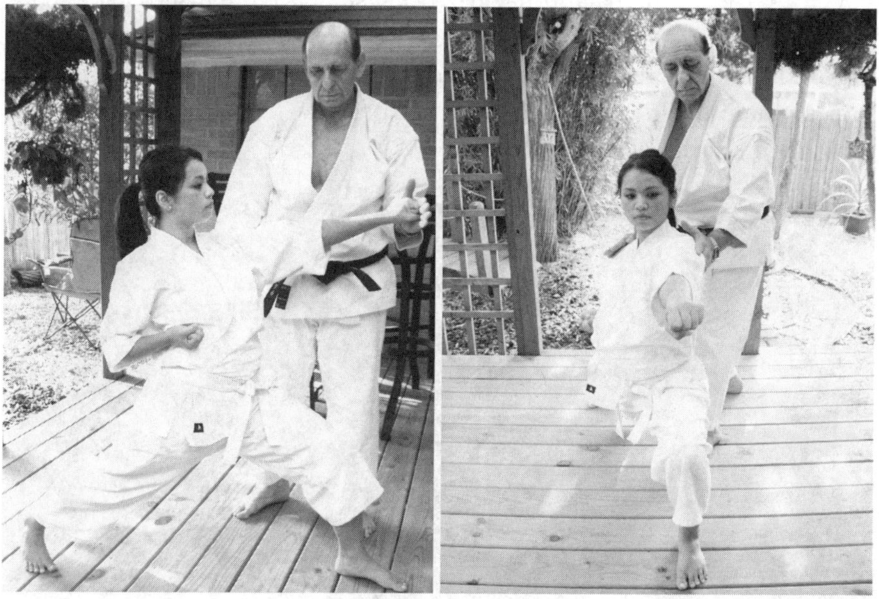

Figure 10: Oi-zuki (incorrect form) and oi-zuki (correct form).

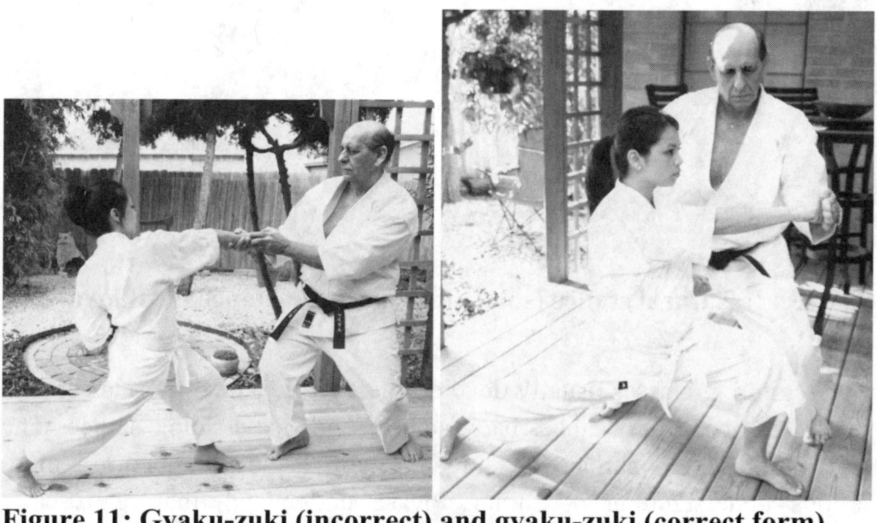

Figure 11: Gyaku-zuki (incorrect) and gyaku-zuki (correct form).

Stances

Karate-Dō Kyōhan lists seven basic stances (tachikata): natural stance (shizentai or hachiji-dachi), front stance (zenkutsu-dachi), back stance (kōkutsu-dachi), horse riding stance (kiba-dachi), cat stance (nekoashi-dachi), feet-together stance (heisoku-dachi), and immovable stance (fudō-dachi).[5] Please refer to chapter 2 of *Kyōhan* for the explanation of these stances.

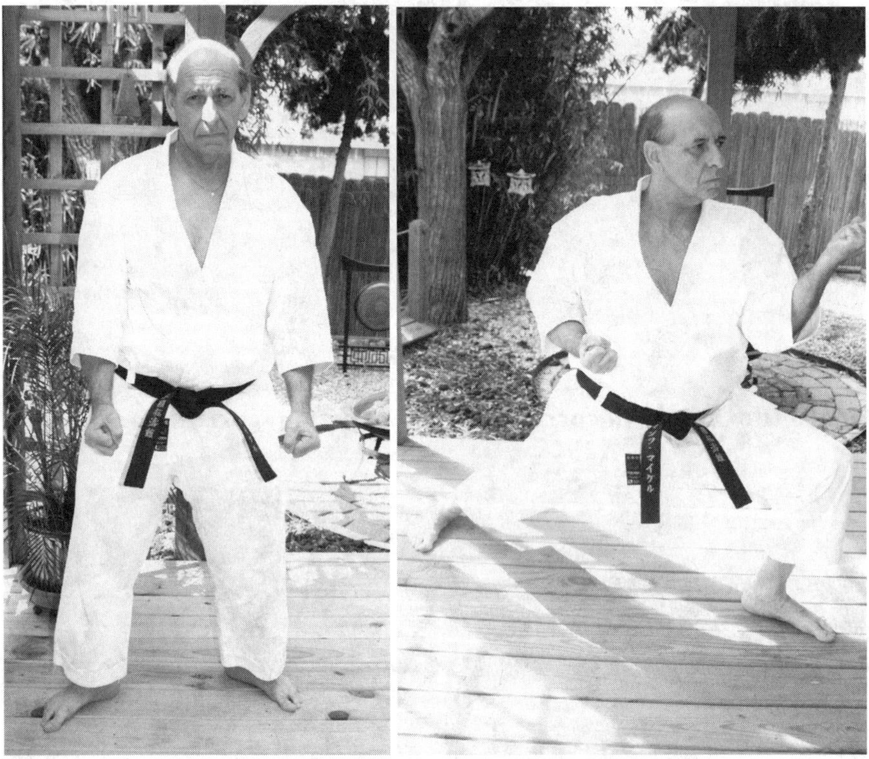

Figure 12: Natural stance (shizentai) and front stance (zenkutsu-dachi).

Beginning classes usually develop the first four of these stances: the natural stance, front stance, back stance, and horse-riding stance. The remaining stances can be developed if you decide to pursue a more serious understanding of karate. Please understand, that realistically karate is not something that is static or fixed. Students often confuse this method of practicing individual techniques as being something that is rigid or something that is hard and unyielding in the application of a technique. The opposite is true. Karate is something that should flow from the body's natural movements with vitality and flexibility.

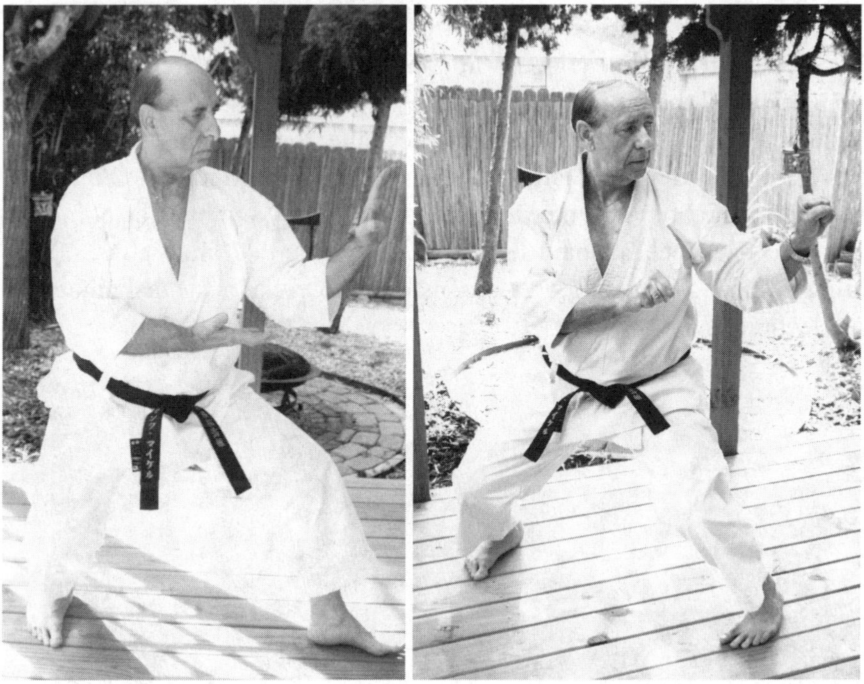

Figure 13: Back stance (kōkutsu-dachi) and horse-riding stance (kiba-dachi).

The stances are designed to build your core and to create the structure for practicing individual techniques. Initially this will be done in place, and then moving forward and backward (in straight-lines).

The study of individual techniques, using fixed or static stances will also help you to gain confidence and a positive mind in building the core elements of practice.

Pulling hand, underarm, elbow, standing leg

At first glance, the above heading seems like four or more separate items. Actually you can look at them as individual items, but when performed together with synchronized unity in conjunction with a technique, they create a "bio-generator" that harnesses and transfers the power of the hips through the karate technique. The trigger or "on-off" switch for this generator is the hikite or what is known as the pulling hand.

The pulling hand, made with a proper fist is pulled back and executed with the fist (fingers up) laid above the hipbone. Making a proper fist and the pulling hand will be covered in Chapter 4 under Hand Techniques. The pulling hand sets the table for the other parts of the "generator" to kick into action. The underarm locks and the elbow hugs the side of the body, all of which are anchored by the back standing leg (with the back heel planted firmly on the ground). Karate power flows through this bio-generator and is transferred to either a fist technique or a foot technique.

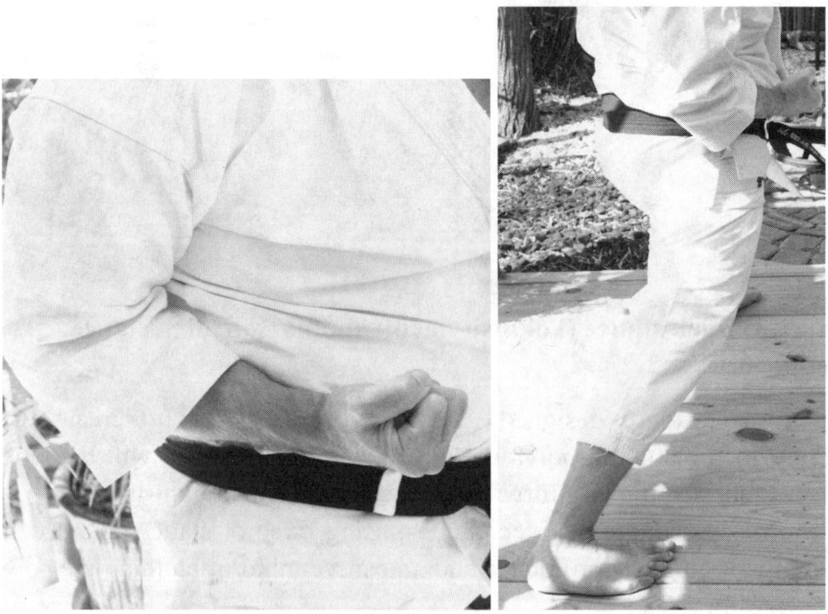

Figure 14: Hikite (pulling hand) and standing leg with the form of the foot and back heel.

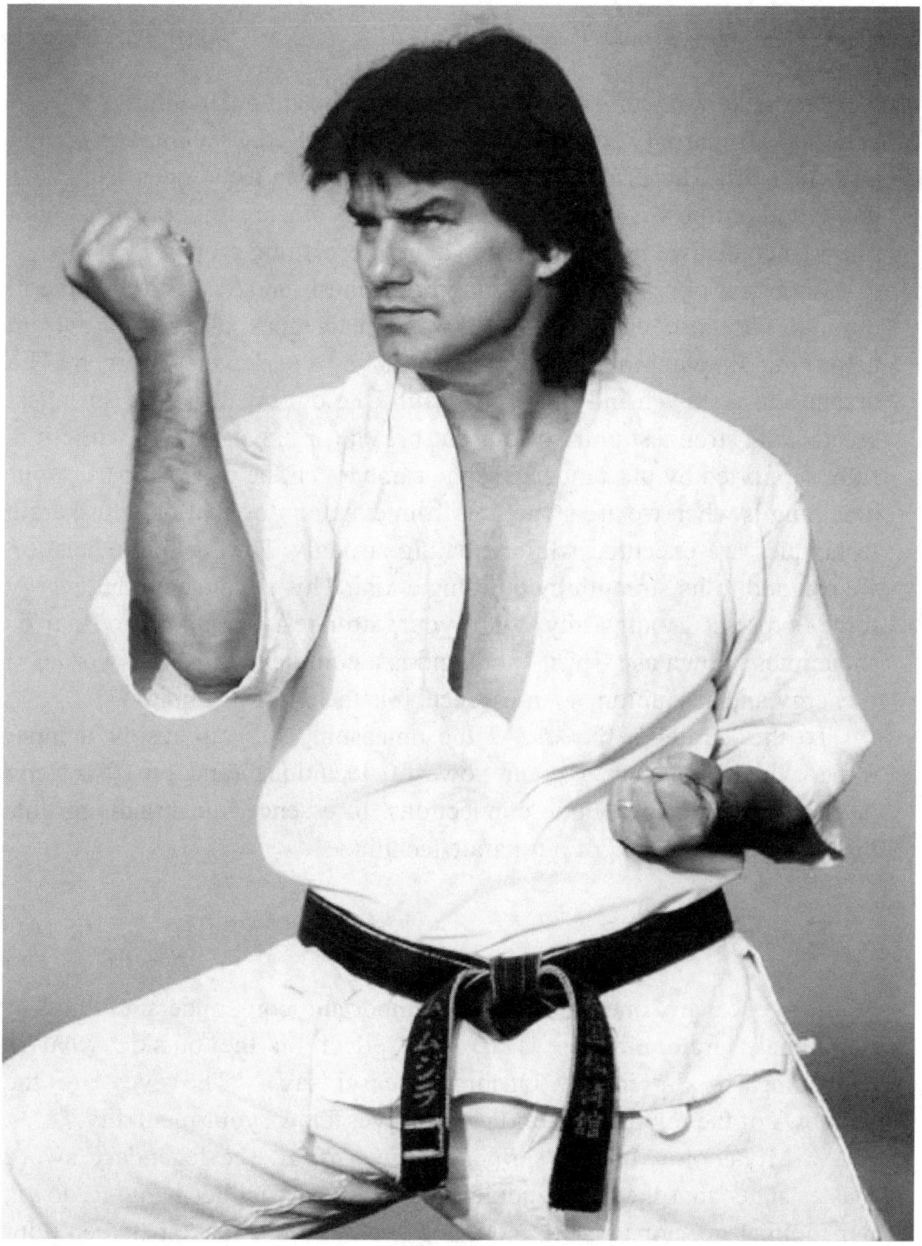

Figure 15: Tom Muzila demonstrates a strong hikite (elbow and underarm).

Breathing

On the surface, this seems like a foolish heading. Breathing? We all breathe. All martial arts have their own waza — the techniques of that particular art. The bridge between our waza (our techniques using our body) and our powerful subconscious mind is our breathing. It is of vital importance that we understand the value of breathing properly.

We begin to practice this strong breathing in mokusō. We breathe in through our nose concentrating on the mechanics of breathing from below our diaphragm supported inwardly by our lower abdomen. The breath out is slower and more powerful. The out-breath is our strongest breath. The strongest point of our out-breath (or exhalation) is while it is fully supported by our tanden. By the same token the weakest part of our breathing is when we are switching from exhaling to inhaling. Our karate techniques are executed while exhaling strongly. During the exhalation we can add to its strength by emitting a kiai. This is your internal energy force expressed outwardly with your strongest breath. The kiai is sometimes known as a spirit shout and is a combination of two words, ki = energy and ai = union, so in essence, it is the energy of union.

To the karate-ka the *kiai* is the unleashing of your resolved inner force, which connects to your powerful technique (and hip) by using proper form and power line connections. In essence, our breathing puts the "icing on the cake" of our karate technique.

Eyes

The eyes are one of the most important core understandings of traditional karate practice. The eyes reflect on the outside what is happening on the inside. Ohshima Sensei says, "The eyes are the windows of the mind. The action of our eyes shows your mentality."[6]

In Miyamoto Musashi's *Book of Five Rings*, the legendary sword master states that the head should be kept erect, "neither hanging down, nor looking up, nor twisted. Your forehead and the space between your eyes should not be wrinkled. Do not roll your eyes nor allow them to blink, but slightly narrow them."[7]

Your eyes should be kept open with your head held level. While practicing basics, always look in the direction of the movement of the technique. In kata practice, your eyes follow your opponent depending on the movements in the form (head straight, eyes penetrating the opponent). During sparring, you must always keep strong eye contact with the opponent. The eyes will reflect the intention of your opponent as it relates to being able to perceive an aggressive attack.

You will soon realize that keeping the head straight with the eyes focused forward helps to create a strong positive mental attitude.

Different types of power

The types of power can be placed into three general categories: thrusting power, snapping power, and swinging power.[8] These types of power can be experienced through the various basic techniques practiced in a beginning class Kinds of power will also be revealed through our practice of katas and in our basic sparring practice. Examples of power include (but not limited to):

- Thrusting — oi-zuki (front punch), gyaku-zuki (reverse punch), yokogeri-kekomi (side-thrust kick).
- Snapping — mae-geri (front kick), yokogeri-keage (side-up kick).
- Swinging — tetsui (hammer fist), mikazuki-geri (crescent kick).

On occasions, the types of power will combine to form a hybrid applied power such as a thrusting technique that has a snapping overtone or a swinging type technique that has a snapping feeling.

Techniques (Waza)

Every martial art has its waza, those techniques that make-up the body of the art. The techniques of karate consist of blocks, strikes, punches, thrusts, and kicks, using all parts of the body. These techniques will be practiced either in a defensive mode or an offensive mode. There are also more subtle forms of waza including torite (escaping), nagewaza (throwing), and kyushu (vital areas of the body). These techniques however are not covered in an introductory class.

The practitioner will use all parts of the body signifying the kara or empty-handed (weaponless) way. This initial stage of practicing techniques is the framework that is coupled with the other core values to build the foundation of the karate structure. However, it should always be understood, that the techniques are just one piece of the puzzle that comprises the dual activity of practicing the dō.

Eventually, a true practitioner understands that the dō must include shin, tai, and waza; that is the spirit or mind, the body, and technique.

Our introduction to practice will build-up the body (tai) through the techniques (waza) and hopefully touch a surface understanding of shin (spirit or mind).

Suggested Reading

Karate-Dō Kyōhan, by Gichin Funakoshi, translated by Tsutomu Ohshima. Chapter 2. Fundamental Elements.

---

[1] Don DePree, Shotokan Karate of America, *Relevance of Karate Practice.*
[2] Tsutomu Ohshima, *Notes on Training*, p. 213.
[3] Tom Muzila, Shotokan Karate of America.
[4] *Ibid.*
[5] Gichin Funakoshi, *Karate-Dō Kyōhan*, pp. 19-20.
[6] Tsutomu Ohshima, *Notes on Training*, p. 212.
[7] Miyamoto Musashi, *A Book of Five Rings*, p. 54.
[8] Tom Muzila, Shotokan Karate of America.

4. Basic Hand Techniques (Te waza)

Study the difference between oi-zuki and gyaku-zuki as a way to learn how to research questions about karate practice.... For me, oi-zuki and gyaku-zuki are like a two-strand rope. Maybe you would say that they are two sides of the same coin. As you attack an opponent, you must be able to use one or the other as the situation requires.[1]

Tsutomu Ohshima
Shihan, Shotokan Karate of America

The basic hand techniques can be divided into blocks, punches, thrusts, and strikes. These techniques are performed either with a closed fist (seiken) or with an open hand (shutō — sword hand or nukite — spear-hand).

Understanding how to make hand techniques requires that you have sufficient skill in making a proper fist or proper open-hand form. A second important concept in executing solid foundational hand techniques is understanding the hikite (pulling hand).

The execution of a proper pulling hand cannot be stressed enough. Your techniques will begin to develop with the understanding of the hikite, as we mentioned in the chapter on core values. The hikite becomes the trigger for your powerful bio-generator to transmit your energy through your technique. We will look at these items individually, and then apply these principals to our basic hand techniques.

There are four basic closed-fist blocks: gedan-barai (down block), ude-uke (inside forearm block), age-uke (rising block), and tetsui-uke (iron hammer block). There is also one basic open hand block: shutō-uke (knife hand block).

There are two basic punches or thrusting techniques: oi-zuki (front punch), gyaku-zuki (reverse punch). These are customarily done with the closed fist; however, one can also make them with a spear-hand. These techniques can also be made with different stances and different types of power. For the initial stage of practicing these techniques, we will focus on the front stance for our four fist blocks and two punches. The open-hand block will be done with the back stance.

Form of Fist and Open Hand

The first order of business for hand techniques is understanding the proper form of the hand when making techniques. Initially we will focus on the fist (seiken) and open hand (shutō/nukite). Please refer to the *Kyōhan* for a detailed description (Chapter 2, pp. 17-19).

The fist simply requires the little finger, ring finger, and middle finger be folded very tightly in against the palm of the hand. The thumb is then wrapped tightly around the index finger (which is also folded in) and the middle finger. The wrist must be held straight, neither forward nor backward.

The open-hand form is made by placing the fingers tightly together (little finger through index finger) and folding the thumb in toward the palm and index finger. The four fingers should create a strong, "bumpy" ridge from the knuckles to the tips.

Please see the diagrams for the forms of the hand as shown on the next page.

1-3. **Making a proper fist** 1.

2.

3. Bottom of fist (tetsui) 3.

4. Regular fist 4.

5. Back fist (uraken) 5.

6-7. **Making proper open hand form**

6. Spear-hand (nukite) 6.

7. Knife hand (shutō) 7.

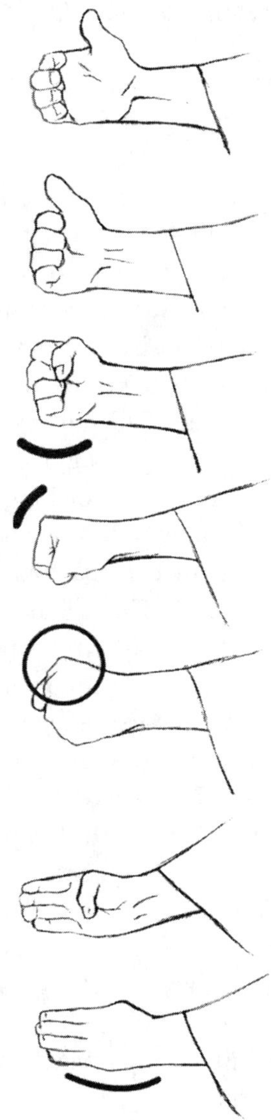

Figure 16: Forms for hand techniques.

Pulling Hand (Hikite)

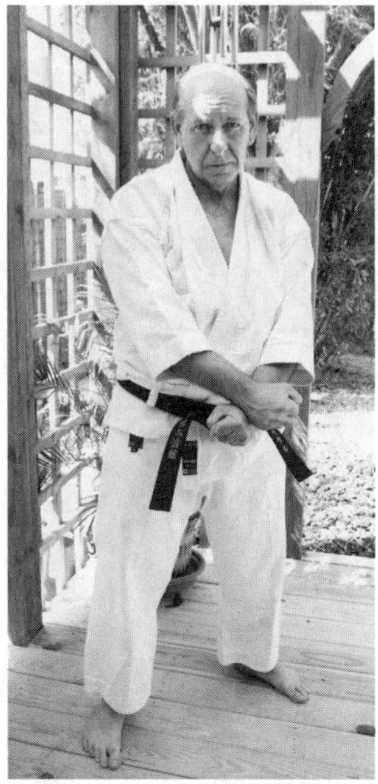

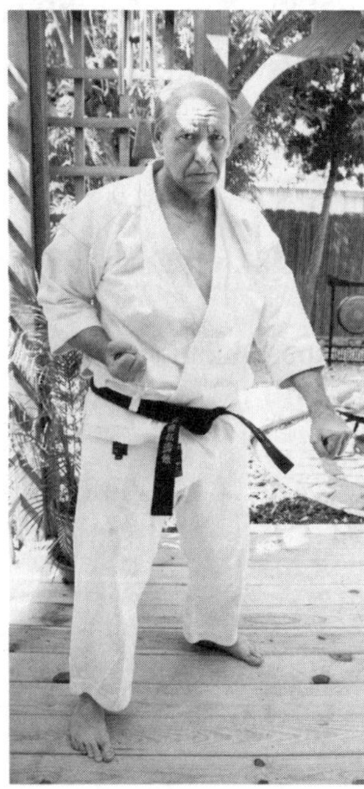

After practicing our fist and open hand we begin to build one of our central core values, the hikite. I have mentioned before that I believe the pulling hand is the trigger for the bio-generator that ties our body together physically to make powerful and penetrating karate techniques. Again this generator consists of our pulling hand, our elbow, our underarm, and our standing leg and back heel. The pulling hand is our switch.

I personally struggled for years trying to find the answer to making better techniques. It was only after about twenty Special Trainings that I realized the value of my pulling hand. The epiphany about my hikite began to change my practice drastically.[2] Therefore, I think it most appropriate to study this from the very beginning of practice. I often heard my seniors talk about this, but somehow I was like Teflon and the concept just kept slipping off. I hope you will catch on to the idea more quickly.

The exercise is to simply stand in a natural stance with the fists crossed in front of the tanden area. (pulling hand fist on top) On command, the pulling hand is drawn powerfully and as exactly as possible to just above the hipbone on the side of the body, elbow in close, underarm tight. The other hand moves slightly in the opposite direction coming to rest even with the opposite standing leg. Please refer to the illustrations.

Making a Punch

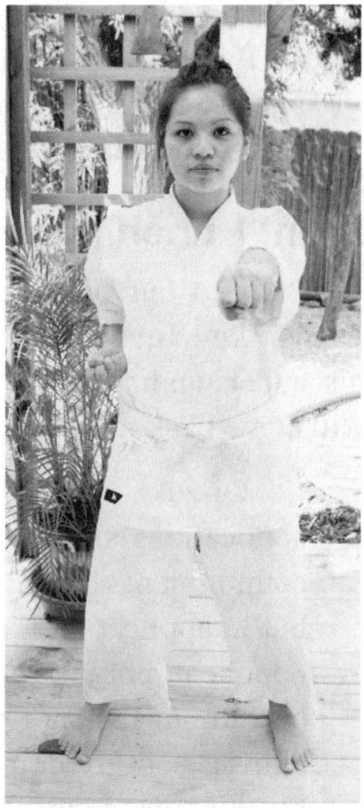

Punches or hand techniques can be made with the fist or open hand. Either can be done with a straight thrusting hip or a turning hip. Our initial development will be the closed fist technique with a thrusting hip.

The training of making a punch (tsuki) is initiated by standing in a natural stance (shizentai). Both feet are firmly planted on the floor with good balance and a solid center of gravity emanating from your tanden area. Next we place one fist on our hipbone with fingers pointed up, the opposite fist (fingers down) is extended at the end of our arm, and is pointed in a straight line directly in front of our body. As the command is given, both arms and fists work in unison as if they were on a taut pulley or bungee cord.

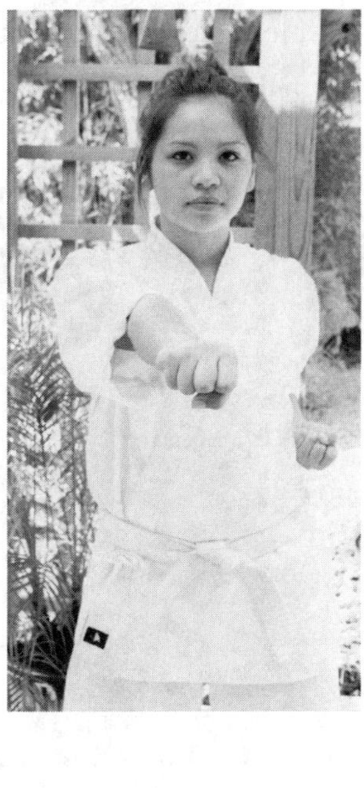

The fist on the hip moves forward in a straight line and, prior to actually punching, rotates in a twisting type of corkscrew motion,[3] ending with the fingers down and back of the hand pointing upward (the knuckles forming a right angle).

Simultaneously, the arm and hand that were extended pull back as if they were on this bungee cord. They make the same twisting motion as they reach the hipbone (fist turning, so the fingers are pointing up.) We have begun the process of learning how to coordinate both sides of the body. (Refer to the *Kyōhan,* chapter 3) and also the illustrations in this chapter.

Punches (Tsuki)

The next phase of punching will be to execute a front punch (oi-zuki) and reverse punch (gyaku-zuki) from a front stance (zenkutsu-dachi).

Front Punch (Oi-zuki)

Prior to our basic discussion of how to execute each technique, I would like to quote Jim Sagawa, one of SKA's top senior instructors, on his understanding of oi-zuki. After learning the technique, I hope you will come back to ponder Mr. Sagawa's insights.

> Oi-zuki embodies elements all other techniques and applications should be based on. Oi-zuki requires bravery and commitment. Its literal translation is "pursuit" of the opponent, but in application it requires breathing and punching through the opponent, not just "at" the opponent. Attempting oi-zuki without best kime [focus of energy] places you in danger, but best kime allows you to dominate your opponent. The most effective blocking is done with the same attitude and much the same movements as oi-zuki.[4]

The front punch will initially be executed standing in place in a front stance, then thrusting the hip forward by stepping in with the back leg.

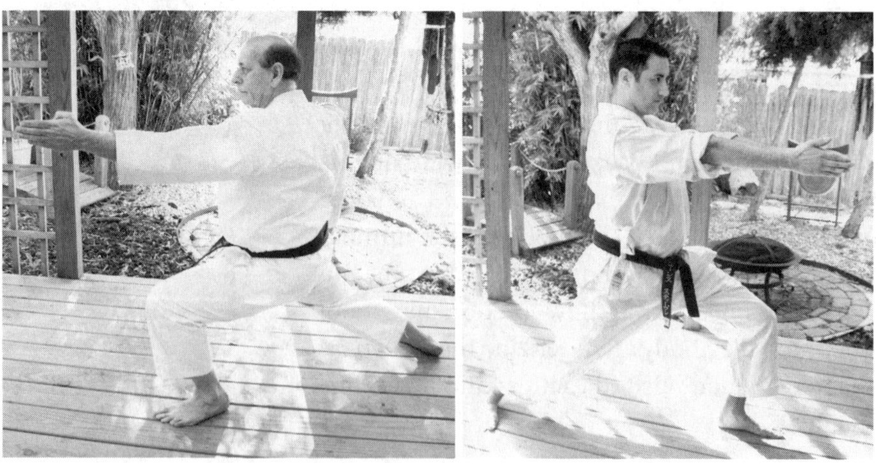

Figure 17: Form for oi-zuki and gyaku-zuki.

Reverse Punch (Gyaku-zuki)

The reverse punch will also be executed in a front stance. However, the stance will be kept stationary and the hand on the hip will be thrust forward. One will immediately notice the shoulders and power lines of this technique and how it differs from the front punch. The final form of the reverse punch will be to have the arm that is opposite the front leg thrust forward. Thus the arm and leg are reversed. This technique is sometimes referred to as a counterpunch because of the quickness in which it can be delivered after blocking an offensive technique. Please review the *Kyōhan* Chapter 3 and the discussion on Ten No Kata Omote in Chapter 7 of this book.

Basic Blocks, Closed Fist

The four basic closed fist blocks are down block (gedan-barai), inside forearm block (ude-uke), rising block (age-uke), and iron hammer block (tetsui-uke).

Down Block (Gedan-Barai)

The down block is a downward sweeping block that has the feeling of a slicing sword. This block is initiated by first standing in a natural stance. (In this instance the blocking arm will be the left arm). The blocking arm is placed with a bent elbow and the closed fist in front of the opposite shoulder (i.e. the left fist in front of the right shoulder). The right arm and fist are held in a straight line over the right leg. (Refer to the pictures on the next page.)

At the command, the left fist sweeps downward across the front of the body. The right fist comes to the hip in a pulling hand. The body remains in a natural stance, but the head and eyes turn to the left in the direction of the block. The blocking arm is straight and ends at the position of the left standing leg within the line of the body. The point is to develop this one-line angular form.

The development of this technique will continue in place by opening your hip sideways (to the left) into a front stance while executing the technique. The final stage in developing this basic block is to make it

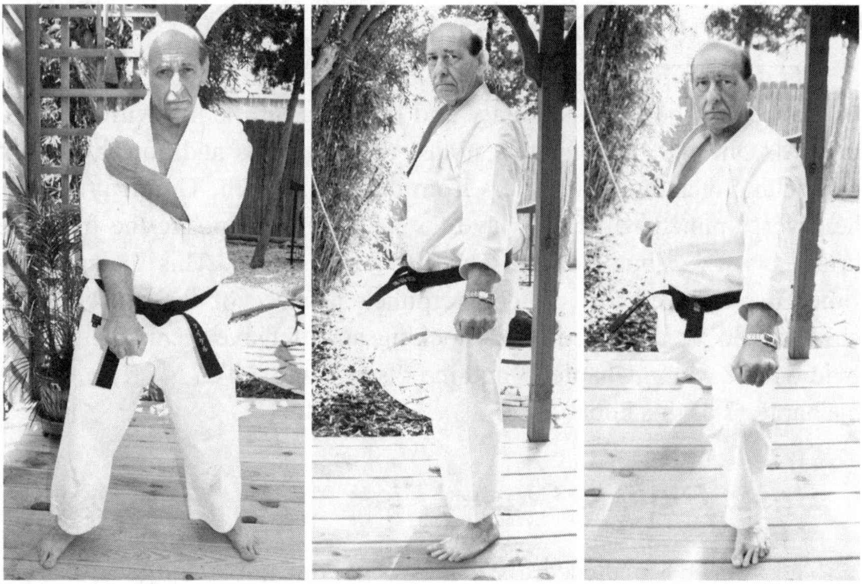

Figure 18: Down block (gedan-barai).

each time we take a step forward in a front stance, usually ten steps before turning around and stepping in the other direction. Moving forward in a front stance will build strong hips and a positive feeling with strong breathing and eyes directed strongly at your opponent.

The later development of this technique will be covered in the chapter on basic sparring. You will learn to apply it as you step back to block an attack coming toward you. It should be noted, however, that we will start from natural stance learning to block to either side. As Ohshima Sensei says,

> We introduce this practice-to-the side to junior members so they can learn to make solid movements to the side, while learning the form of basics. Then after learning moving to the side very well, they can make the same form stepping forward.... I have found that people can move their hips to the side much more easily than stepping forward.[5]

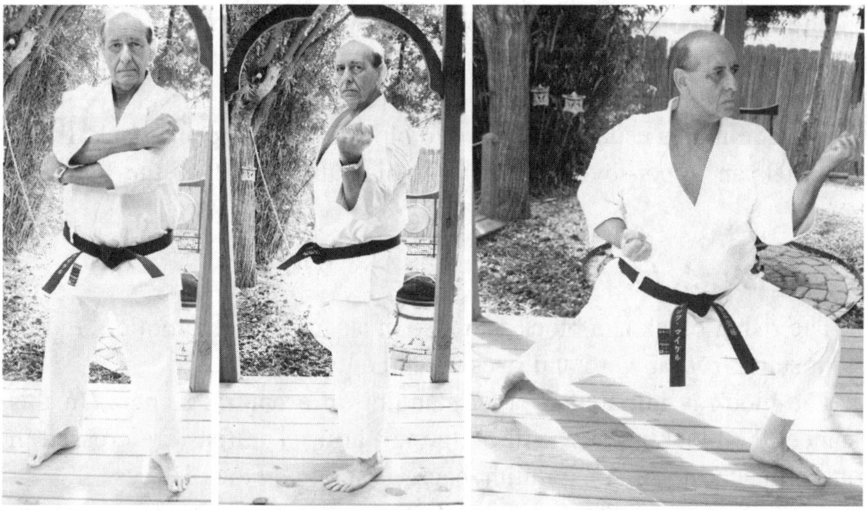

Figure 19: Inside forearm block (ude-uke).

Inside Forearm Block (Ude-Uke)

The inside forearm block moves in a semi-circular motion from inside to outside.

This block is initiated by first standing in a natural stance. (In this instance the blocking arm will be the left arm). The blocking arm is placed with a closed fist under the elbow of the right arm. Both are crossed in front of the body, as shown in the pictures.

At the command, the left arm moves in a semi-circular motion to the left. The right fist comes to the hip in a pulling hand. The body remains in a natural stance, but the head and the eyes turn to the left in the direction of the block. The blocking arm is bent and the fist ends up about shoulder height. The left wrist is slightly bent outward with the fingers pointing back towards you. The elbow should be in line with the body about a fist's distance from the side of the body. The underarm is tight. The front knee, fist, shoulder, hip, and back leg are all along the same line.

The development of this block continues in place by opening the hip sideways (to the left) into a front stance while executing the technique.

The final stage, as in down block, is to make the block while moving forward in a front stance. Please refer to the down block for further explanations on the progression of developing the block.

The ude-uke is usually designed to block a middle level attack. It can also block an upper-level attack by raising the height of the blocking arm.

Rising Block (Age-Uke)

The rising block is a block that also in a semi-circular motion. In this case it starts from inward and rises up and outward.

The block is initiated by first standing in a natural stance. (In this instance, the blocking arm will be the left arm.) The fists are crossed in front of the chest, fingers pointing back, as shown in the pictures.

At the command, the left and right fists make a ripping-apart motion. The right fist goes to the hip in a pulling hand and the left fist makes a semi-circular motion (inward-out) starting in front of the mouth area, past the nose, and lifting up and out. The arm turns outward in a repelling action. The arm creates a right angle, with the left eye fixed on the inside of the left elbow. The right eye looks under the arm, which is extended on an angled line past the forehead. The elbow is always kept inside the line of the body.

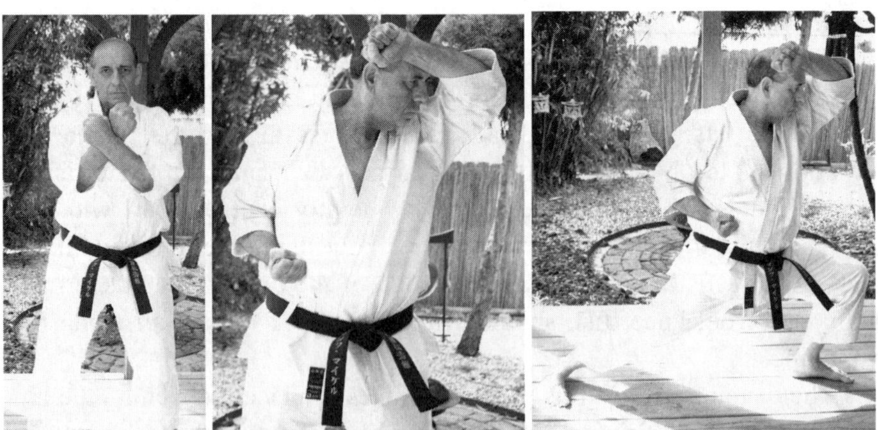

Figure 20: Rising block (age-uke).

The development of this technique will continue in place by opening the hip sideways (to the left) into a front stance while executing the technique. The final stage in developing this basic block is to make it as we step forward in a front stance. Please refer to the down block for further explanations on the progression of developing the rising block.

The age-uke is designed to block an upper-level attack at the face.

Hammer Block (Tetsui-Uke)

Tetsui is also known as hammer fist. It can also be referred to as uchikomi. The tetsui fist is the fleshy portion on the little-finger side of the hand. Usually, when using the hammer block (whether blocking or striking) a turning hip is employed.

Therefore, as we practice this technique, we will not create the same one-line feeling to the side as we used with the other blocks. Instead, we will practice the dynamics of making a turning hip, both forward and backward.

We begin standing in a natural stance with our hands on our hips with the elbows extended outward (akimbo). At the command, turn your hips in a circular motion toward the front first with one side and then the other. This will give you the feeling of turning your hips when you make a technique. It should be noted, that the elbows are extended only for the purpose of this drill. Otherwise, elbows will always remain inside the line of the body.

Once we have a feeling for turning the hip, we begin to practice this block in place. The blocking arm is raised above the head so the elbow is above the shoulder and the forearm in vertical with the hammer or tetsui fist pointed forward. For the most part the elbow is within the body's line relative to your opponent. This will relax the shoulder and hence will not weaken your technique. The opposite fist can be brought up in a vertical line, right in front of the nose and mouth. On command, the blocking arm is dropped in a downward motion across the face, coming to rest in front of the opposite shoulder (fingers pointing in). The opposite fist is drawn strongly back to the hip making a powerful pulling hand. This movement creates a turning hip. The more relaxed you are when initiating this technique, the more dynamic it becomes. (Refer to the pictures.)

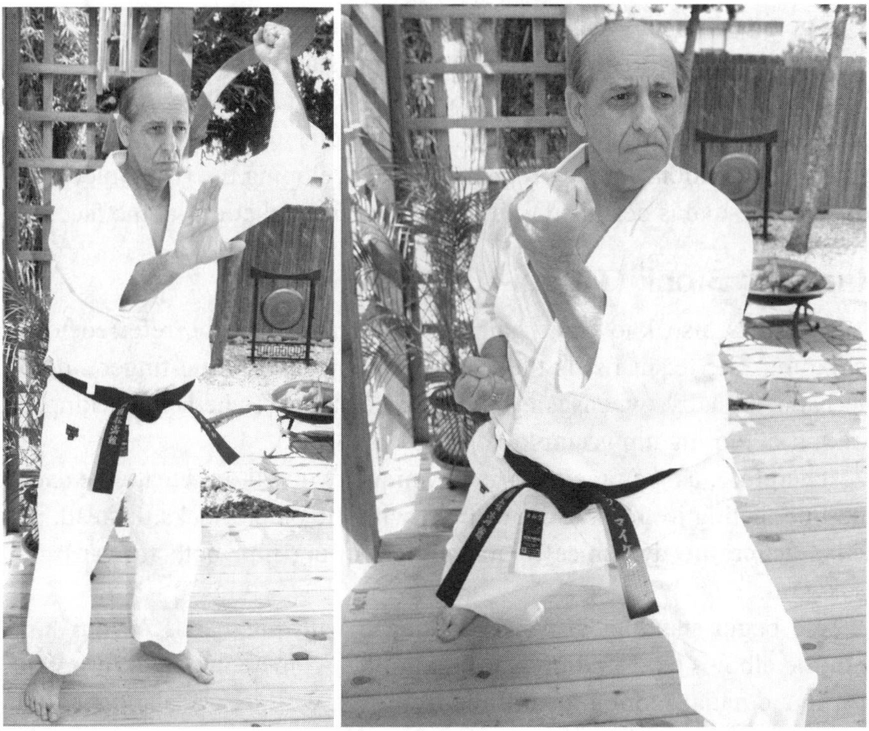

Figure 21: Hammer block (tetsui-uke).

Continuing with the development of this block, you make the same technique as you step into a front stance. For example, standing in a natural stance, the right arm is raised in preparation to block. The left arm is raised in front of the body. On command, the right leg steps forward into a front stance, while the right arm delivers the striking block. The left fist is pulled to the hip as a hikite.

The next stage of this block is to apply it stepping in a front stance. Please refer to the down block for further explanations on the progression of developing the block.

Basic Blocks, Open Hand

The last basic block is an open hand block called the shutō-uke, the knife-hand block. Please refer to Figure 16 at the beginning of this chapter and to *Karate-Dō Kyōhan* for more detail on the mechanics of making the proper form with the hand and fingers.

This block, along with the first three closed fist blocks can be developed using a one-line feeling by opening the hip sideways.

Knife Hand Block (Shutō-Uke)

The shutō-uke or knife hand block is customarily made with back stance (kōkutsu-dachi). During the initial stage of developing this block, we will make it with a natural stance.

This block is initiated, by standing in a natural stance. (In this instance, the blocking arm will be the left arm).

At the command, the eyes turn left, the blocking hand (left) will be placed next to the right ear (elbow remains inside the body's line). The right arm extends horizontally across and under the solar plexus area. This arm should protect the middle-level area of your body, also forming a type of pulling hand with your elbow close to your body and your underarm slightly tight. As you turn to the left with your eyes, the body remains half-facing, but the right foot and leg turn slightly toward the left to create a strong back leg connection. The block cuts from the ear down across the body coming to rest in line with the front standing leg. The

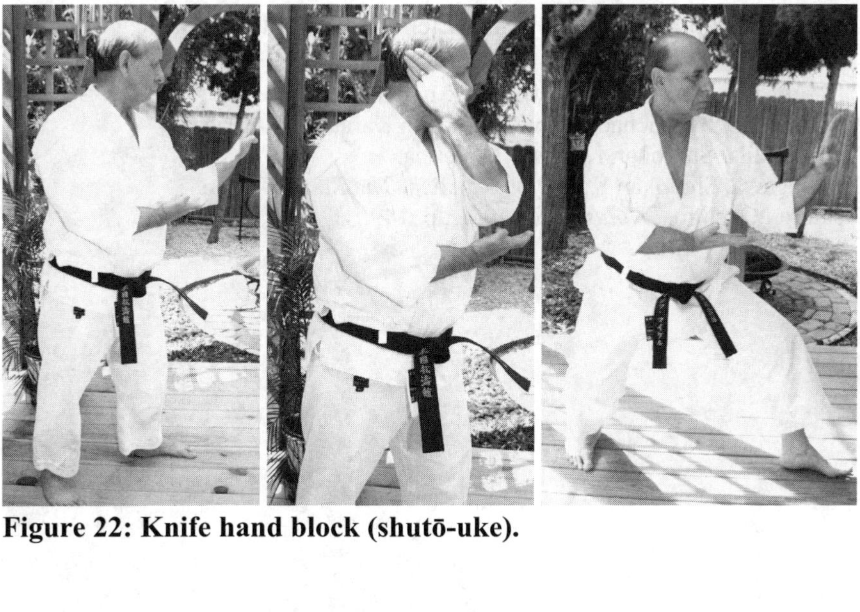

Figure 22: Knife hand block (shutō-uke).

blocking arm is bent at a right angle and is in line with your body. The elbow should never stick out from the body's line relative to your opponent. Refer to the pictures above.

The next stage of development will be to make the same movements as described above, but to make them using back stance. When practicing the technique in back stance, it is imperative that you develop a stance that not only moves away from the opponent's technique, but also can resist the pushing onslaught of the opponent. In other words you must have a strong foundational back leg.

The shutō-uke is next made by stepping-back from a natural stance with one leg, returning to a natural stance, stepping back with the other leg, and returning again to natural stance. This is a more realistic application of this technique, which can be practiced stepping straight back or stepping back on an angle.

The final stage can be made in marching mode, both forward and then stepping back. As mentioned in the section on the down-block, the further development of this technique will show how it is applied in sparring.

Suggested Reading

Karate-Dō Kyōhan by Gichin Funakoshi, translated by Tsutomu Ohshima. Chapter 2. Fundamental Elements, Chapter 3. Basic Training.

---

[1] Tsutomu Ohshima, *Notes on Training*, pp. 101-102.
[2] Commentary by Michael Mantz, Shotokan Karate of America.
[3] Tom Muzila, Shotokan Karate of America.
[4] Jim Sagawa, Shotokan Karate of America, *The Road to Irimi.*
[5] Tsutomu Ohshima, *Notes on Training*, p. 149.

5.
Basic Kicking Techniques (Ashi-Waza)

Kicks are a special feature of Karate against other martial arts, so our legs have to be strong enough to destroy opponents with kicks and stamps. The strongest part of any kick has to be the standing leg. Whenever you execute a kick, your standing leg supports not only the weight of your whole body but also your opponent's power and weight.[1]

Tsutomu Ohshima
Shihan, Shotokan Karate of America

The basic kicking techniques that will be covered are front kick (mae-geri), round kick (mawashi-geri), side-up kick (yokogeri-keage), side-thrust kick (yokogeri-kekomi), crescent kick (mikazuki-geri), and stamping kick (fumikomi).[2]

Foundational Concepts

There are certain foundational concepts that you must develop when studying kicking techniques. The most important of these concepts is the standing leg. We must also have an understanding of the movement and positioning of the hips, arms, knees, and the form of the feet when the

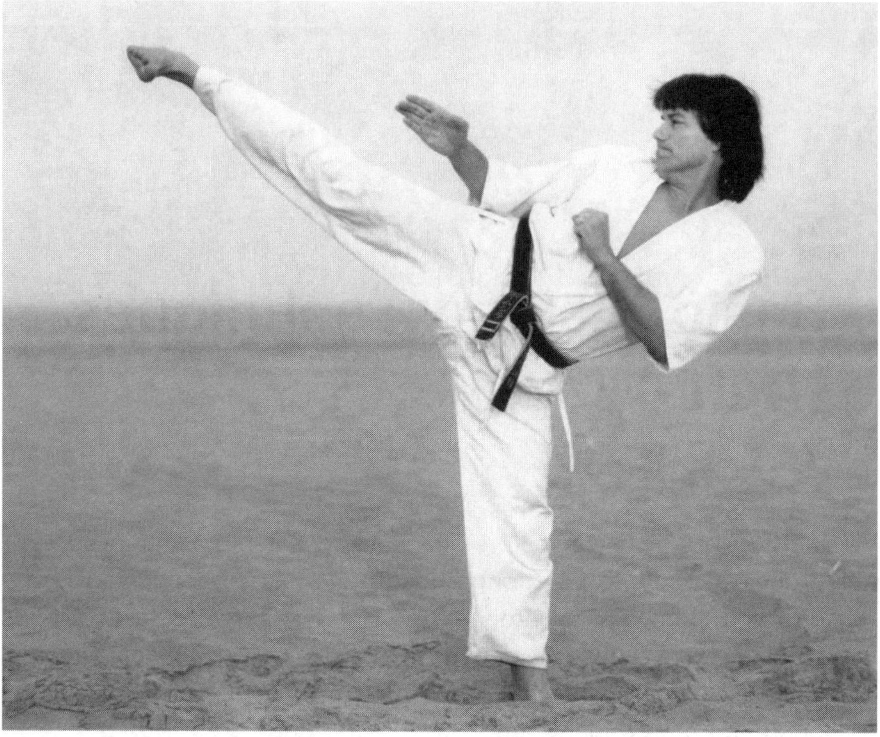

Figure 23: Tom Muzila making yokogeri-kekomi using a strong standing leg.

kick is delivered. These concepts combine together to generate a powerful hip-centered kick.

Standing Leg

Kicking techniques force us to stand on one leg while we kick with the other. The leg that we stand on has to be strong enough to support the weight of our body. We also have to be balanced. Add to that the actual karate technique and the movement and strength of the opponent. Combining all of these factors, it is evident that the standing leg must form a powerful base.

Hips

Kicks can be made with a hip moving straight forward, a turning hip, or a side-to-side hip. Each kick has its own hip movement, but the basic concept of a hip that provides power by connecting the standing leg and the kicking leg is there in each of the kicks.

Arms and Elbows

Kicking basically takes place from the waist downward. The arms should not be lifted or moved upward or outward while making our kicks. The elbows should also stay inside our body's line. The arm that remains with the standing leg for most of the kicks (mikazuki-geri is slightly different) becomes a type of stabilizer that helps anchor a strong standing leg. So in essence, we form a strong standing side consisting of a strong leg with a securely planted foot and heel and an elbow tucked close to the body with a slightly tightened underarm.

Knees

The proper mechanical movement of the knees is vital to executing an effective kicking technique. For front kick, side-thrust kick, and stomping kick the knee initially should be raised to the chest. A knee raising drill should be practiced so you develop the habit of raising the knee when kicking.

The drill consists of standing in a front stance or modified front stance and raising the back knee forward to touch the chest. As the back leg moves forward, it is brought very close to the front standing leg brushing against the front standing leg. It continues until the knee touches the chest. The knee and foot are then returned to their original position.

Other kicks also have proper initial locations for the knee, as we will see in the individual descriptions.

Feet and Toes

The six basic kicking techniques consist of three snapping kicks, two thrusting kicks, and one swinging or sweeping kick. The elementary form of the toe or foot when actually delivering these kicks will be the ball of the foot, the side edge (blade), the heel, and the flat side or bottom arch of the foot. When applying a kicking technique, the toe, heel, or contact portion of the foot should be pointed toward and into the opponent (not away or upward) creating power that drives through.

Front Kick (Mae-geri)

The front kick can be done with snapping or, sometimes, thrusting power. Our beginning practice will focus on snapping power. Our basic front kick will also be made by striking with the ball of the foot.

Already having practiced raising the knee, we will practice this kick with certain basic core elements: strong standing leg, light kicking leg, square hips, and elbows in. We can create a front kick drill by positioning our hips in the final square form prior to executing a completed kick. (See the pictures on the beginning drill.)

For the drill we stand with square hips almost in a feet-together

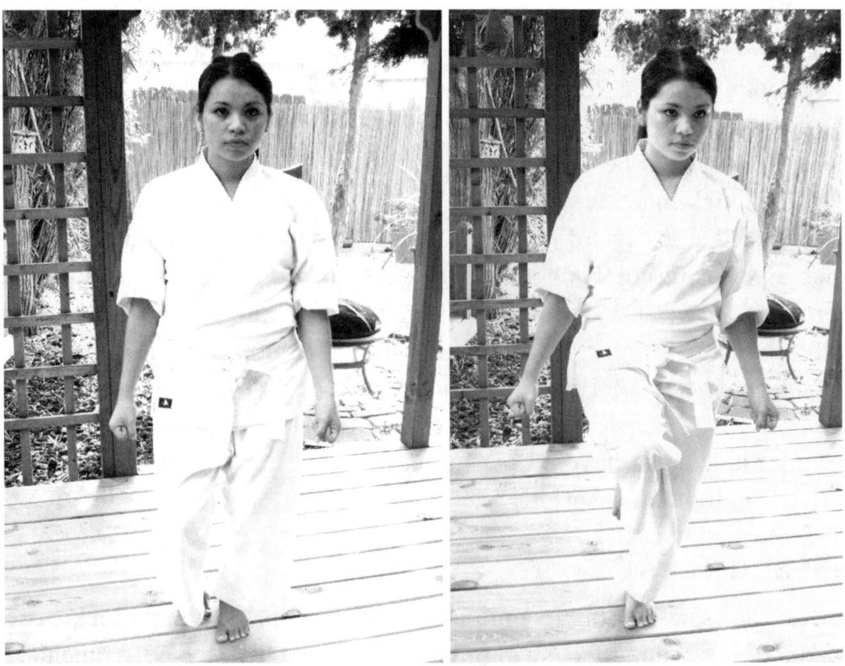

Figure 24: Beginning front kick drill.

stance (heisoku-dachi). The right leg is slightly bent and placed a little behind the left, resting on the ball of the foot or toes. The left foot is solidly planted as a strong standing leg. As the command is given, the right knee is lifted, coming very close to the left leg, and snapped upward and outward. Then it is brought back and returned to its original position.

The feel is to have a light kicking leg and a strong standing leg with powerful square hips prior to the forward movement. There is also a sensation of the hips rolling or turning over. To help stabilize our arms/elbows, five-pound weights may be held in each hand and held against the side of the body. The weights will help keep the arms from moving. They will also help keep the elbows close to the body.

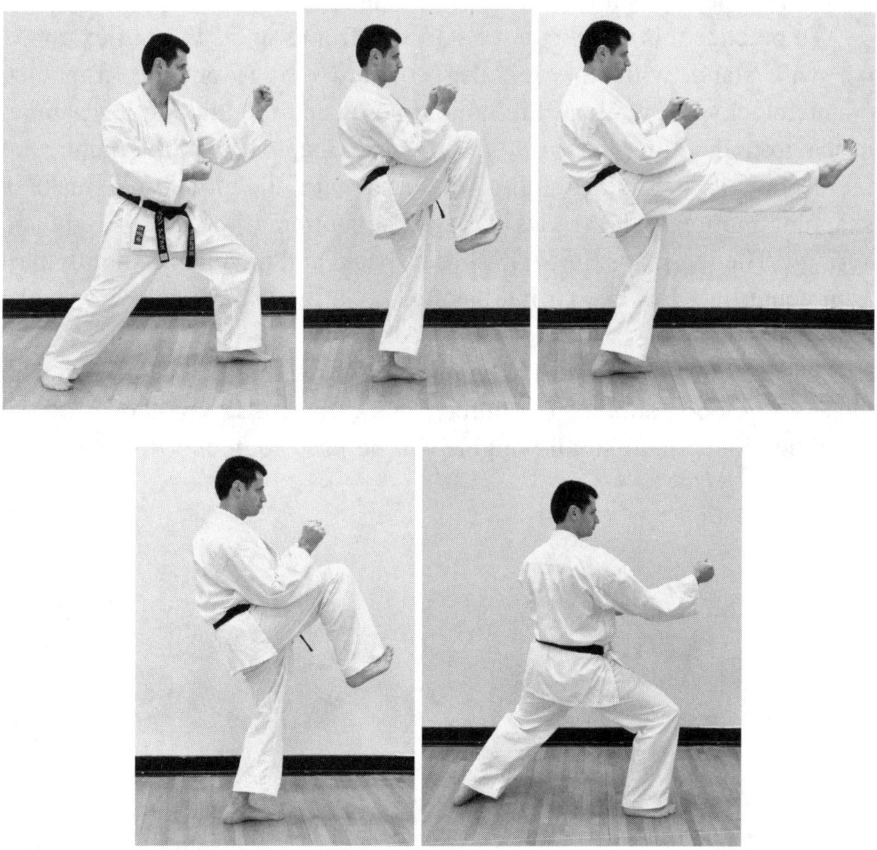

Figure 25: Stepping front kick (mae-geri).

This exercise can be followed by making kicks from a front stance in place, and finally moving forward repeating one technique after the other. The kicking leg is light and quick and the standing leg and side are anchored and powerful.

Round Kick (Mawashi-Geri)

The round kick, sometimes called the roundhouse kick, is made with a rotating hip. This kick is made with a snapping power and, as a basic study, we will use the ball of the foot as our contact area. The key elements to practice are the standing or pivoting leg, anchoring arm, position of the leg as it rises, and follow-through.

To practice this technique we start in a front stance. For our example, we will stand with the left leg forward. Pivot on the front leg counterclockwise, while at the same time raising the kicking leg parallel to the ground. (Refer to *Karate-Dō Kyōhan* Chapter 3 and the pictures of the technique below). As the hip turns with the pivot leg, make a snapping motion with the kicking leg. The motion of the kick is light and springy. The leg snaps the kick, springs back, and then lands slightly past your centerline. Before starting the next kick, move the front leg to make a front stance.

The elbow and arm that remain with the standing leg should be kept close to the body similar to a hikite. This creates a strong anchor on the standing side. Again small weights can be used to anchor the arms and elbows.

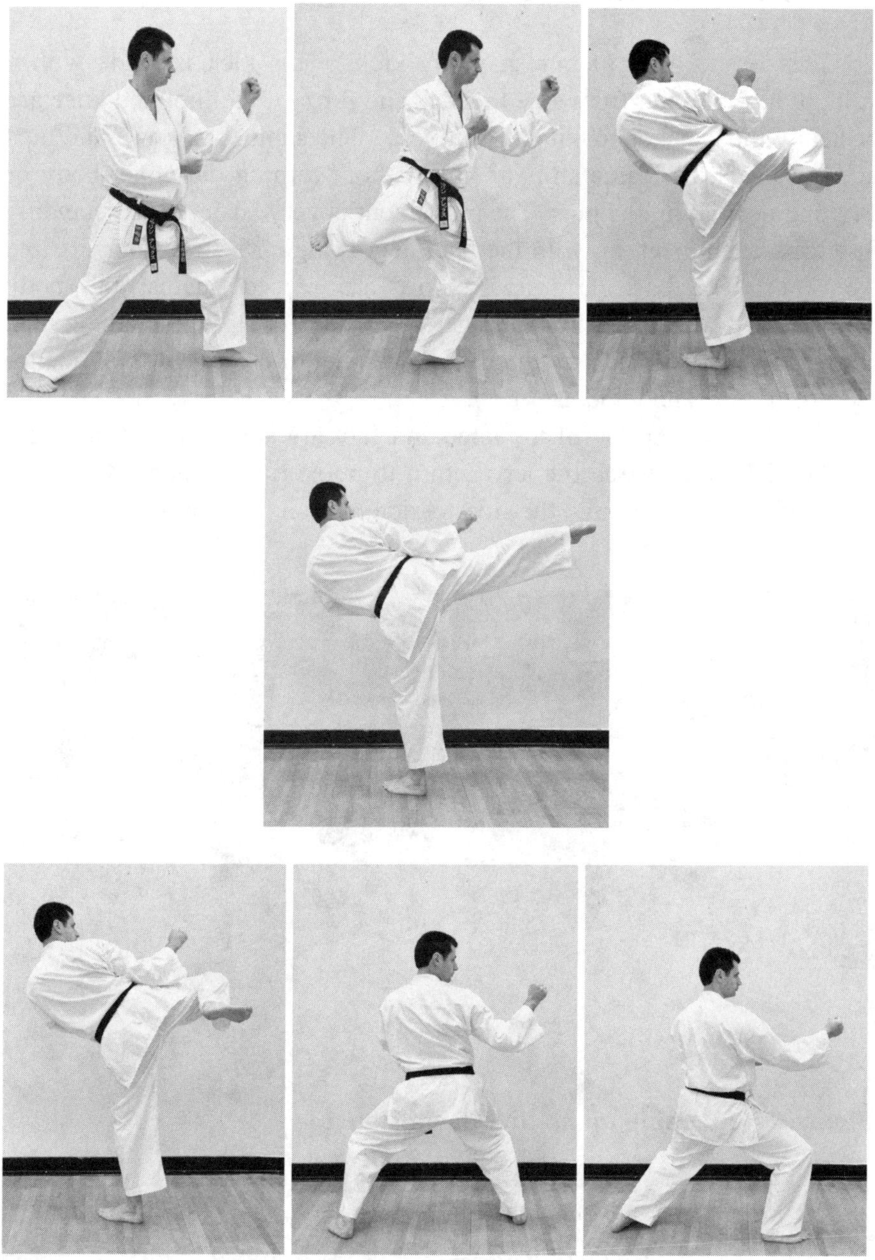

Figure 26: Round kick (mawashi-geri).

Side-up Kick (Yokogeri-Keage)

This is the third of our snapping kicks. This kick is made with a straight hip, moving from side to side. The form of the foot and knee are basically the same as making a front kick. The shoulders, knee, and hips need to be on the same straight line without turning the upper-body or twisting or rotating the hips. The movement is very basic. While standing in a kiba-dachi, step up with the back leg, bringing it to rest against the front leg. The back arm and elbow are placed against the body connecting with the back standing leg, forming a strong standing side. (Refer to the discussion on the use of weights to create a strong anchor with the elbow and underarm.)

The kicking motion of the knee and foot are similar to a front kick. As the kick is delivered the legs return to horse riding stance. The body faces sideways all through the side-to-side motion of the hips.

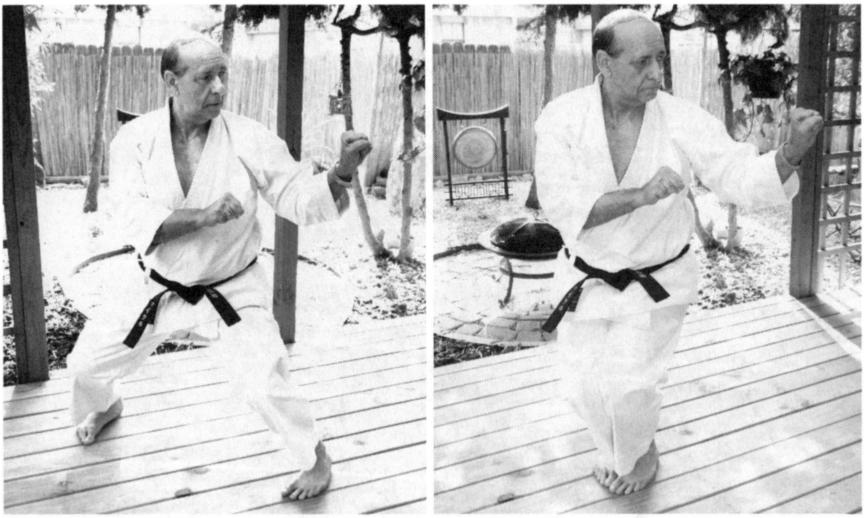

Figure 27: Stepping up in kiba-dachi stance.

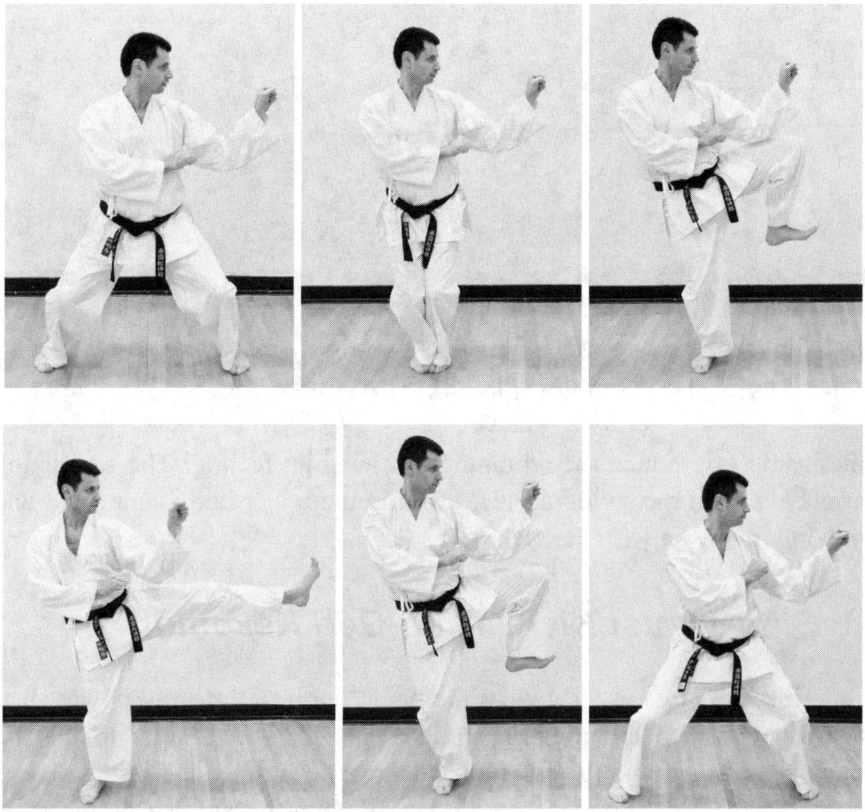

Figure 28: Side-up kick (yokogeri keage).

Crescent Kick (Mikazuki-Geri)

This kick is neither a thrusting nor snapping technique, but is executed with more of a swinging or sweeping feeling. The form of the foot and leg are actually the same basic motion made for a foot sweeping technique. The striking portion of the foot is the flat portion of the bottom of the foot. It can also be made with the outer blade of the foot.

The crescent kick is a natural swinging motion of the leg. It is a kick that can be made fairly easily and can be realistically applied in a natural motion against the opponent's knee or thigh. This kick is made with a turning hip from a horse riding stance. The knee is unlocked, turning to

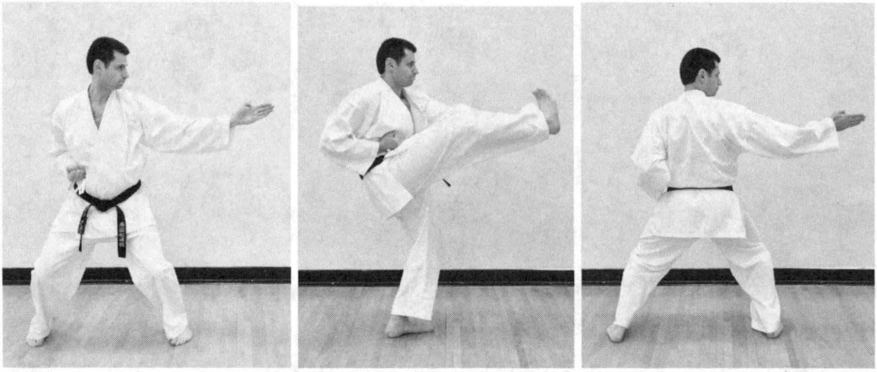

Figure 29: Crescent kick (mikazuki geri).

the inside to produce the whipping or swinging feeling. The stabilizing arm stays with the swinging leg, keeping the upper body connected and moving in unison with the kick.

Side-Thrust Kick (Yoko-Geri Kekomi)

This kick uses exactly what the name implies, thrusting power. It is also done with a hip moving straight side to side (similar to the hip movement in side-up kick). If executed properly, the side-thrust kick is probably the most powerful kick that we have. It can also be the most difficult to learn. The initial movement of the legs and arm is the same as side-up kick. Standing in a horse riding stance, step up with the back leg, bringing it to rest exactly against the front leg. The back elbow and underarm are firmly placed against the body as shown in the pictures. The kicking (front) knee is raised and, together with the heel of the foot, clears the body as both are being raised up and out. The heel does not move behind the hip. The bent knee is then straightened as it is thrust outward creating a straight line with the heel of the kicking leg and the heel of the standing leg. The anchoring arm is held close to the body to create a stabilizer. This is especially important for this kick. One has a feeling of thrusting with the hip as well as the leg and foot.

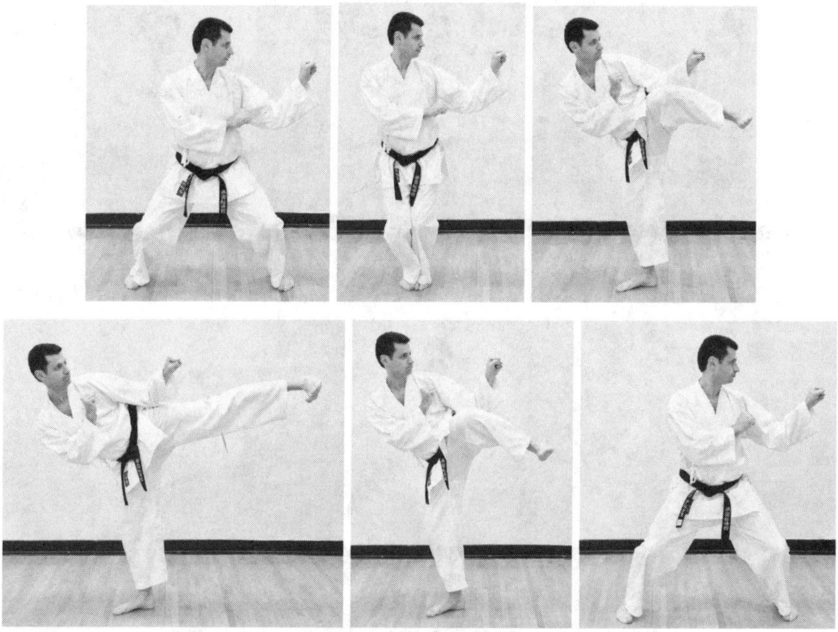

Figure 30: Side-thrust kick (yokogeri-kekomi).

It is important to make sure that the knee (with heel) that is preparing to kick clears the body, otherwise the motion will create something other than a thrust kick (probably a roundhouse kick).

Stamping Kick (Fumikomi)

Fumikomi is the last basic kick. It has a thrusting power very much like the side-thrust kick. The form of the stamping kick has the same foundational movement as the side-thrust kick. The standing leg and anchor arm are very important in developing a powerful thrusting motion with the kicking leg and hip.

The initial practice form is made from a natural stance. Step forward with one leg into a front stance. While stepping forward to kick, the eyes and head turn in the direction of the kick. (When stepping in with the left leg, the head and eyes would turn to the right.)

The rear leg and foot are lifted to the chest and thrust downward toward the opponent, targeting the thigh, knee, shin, ankle, or instep. As

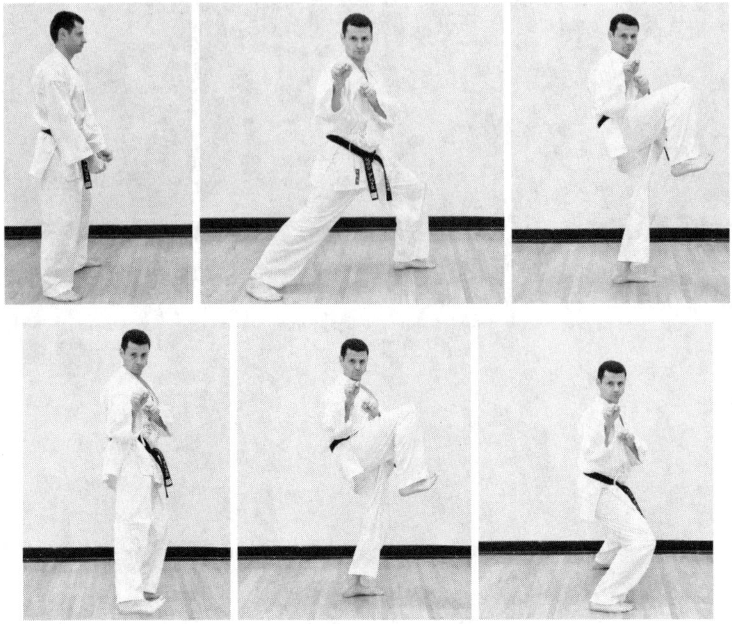

Figure 31: Stamping kick (fumikomi)

the kick is made, the kicking heel, thigh, upper body, and head form a straight alignment which creates a powerful thrusting motion. The standing leg is bent slightly with the elbow and underarm of the anchor arm held close to the body creating a strong standing side.

After the kick is completed, step back to a natural stance in the original location. The motion is then repeated on the other side.

This kick is powerful and very natural, especially during close combat with the opponent. I think it is also a very useful self-defense technique for women (when they learn to execute it properly).

Suggested Reading

Karate-Dō Kyōhan by Gichin Funakoshi, translated by Tsutomu Ohshima. Chapter 2. Fundamental Elements, pp. 23-26 (Foot Techniques), Chapter 5. Kicking Matches, pp. 220-222.

---

[1] Tsutomu Ohshima, *Notes on Training*, p. 118.

[2] Gichin Funakoshi, *Karate-Dō Kyōhan*, pp. 23-26.

6.
Basic Forms (Katas)

> Katas hold crystals of knowledge which are passed down from senior to junior.... We must remember clearly that each movement has to be realistic. We cannot make changes or exaggerate movements in the katas to impress the general public. Instructors have to make sure each movement in the kata conforms to Master Funakoshi's textbook and is executed exactly as Master says.[1]
>
> *Tsutomu Ohshima*
> *Shihan, Shotokan Karate of America*

Generally, a kata is a form that has offensive and defensive techniques. These techniques are done within a certain line of movement (embusen).[2] The movements of a kata are also executed with a predetermined rhythm or flow, using the cardinal points described by Master Funakoshi: expansion and contraction of the body, slow and fast movement of the body, and light and heavy application of strength.[3]

In the discussion on the history and development of karate, Master Funakoshi suggested that there is really only one karate with two distinct schools or training methods: Shōrin and Shōkei. The first edition of *Karate-Dō-Kyōhan* divides the Shotokan katas into these two schools.

Shōrin katas are light and quick with rapid movements back and forth. The Shōkei katas are the opposite. They are powerful and forceful with stronger and thicker movements than the Shōrin katas. The Master

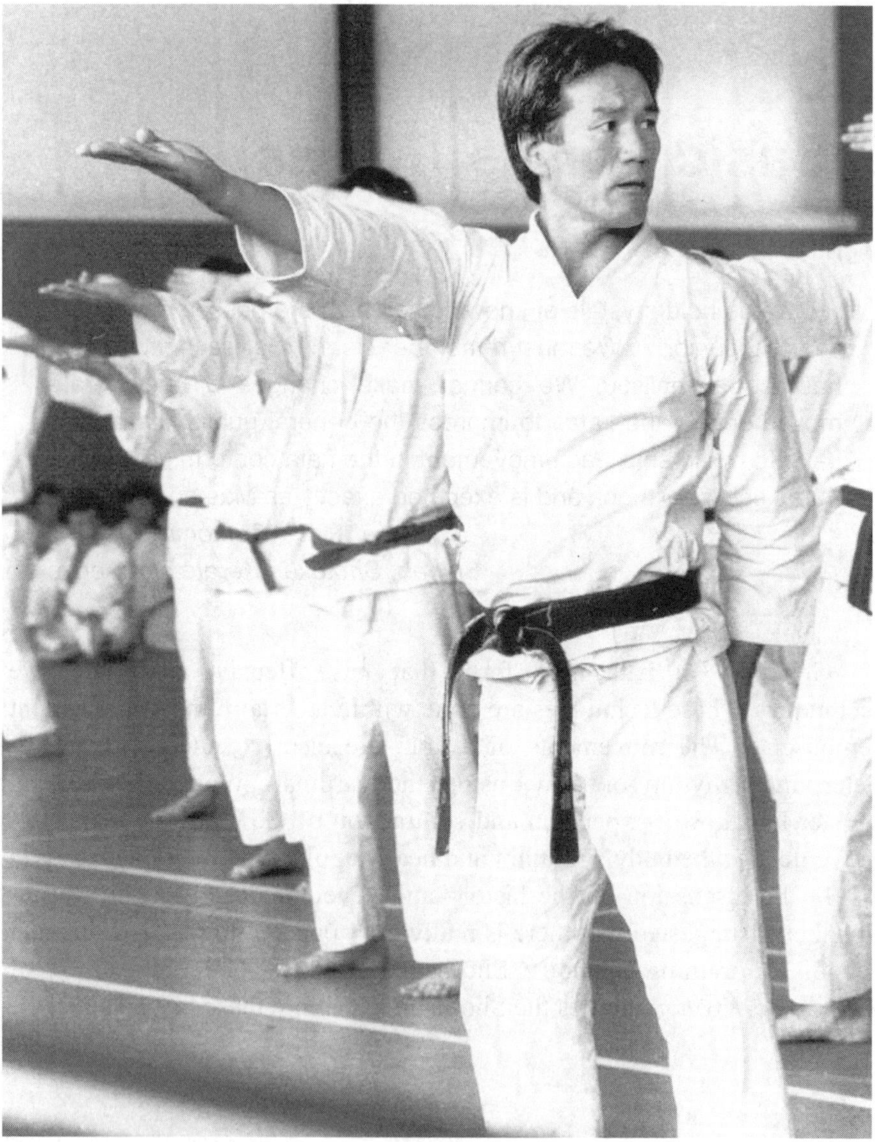

Figure 32: Ohshima Sensei teaching kata.

felt that both of these schools have their strengths and weaknesses, one not being superior to the other. Master Funakoshi was very instrumental in teaching both forms of katas[4] and eventually selected nineteen katas as the basis for his Shotokan teaching. (These nineteen katas are displayed in *Karate-Dō Kyōhan* as translated by Tsutomu Ohshima.)

Katas should also be performed with a sense of being prepared or vigilant in relation to an opponent. This feeling should carry all the way through the form. Your breathing must be coordinated with balanced, dynamic physical movements. In other words, you should practice to attain good mental and physical balance.

Other points to remember when you practice katas are getting ready at the beginning of the kata (yoi), returning to the ready stance at the end of the kata (yame), and paying attention to the target that a particular technique has been designed to strike or block. Katas should be practiced as originally designed. Don't change the movements or rhythm of the form.

Saying this a different way, katas are like the forms every martial art uses to teach you lessons experts discovered in the past. The art of karate is no different than any other martial art in that it creates a method of practice through these forms that help you assimilate techniques and creatively apply them in realistic combat situations.

I will not attempt to give pictures of the moves in the katas. This has already been done by Ohshima Sensei in his translation of the first edition of Master Funakoshi's *Karate-Dō Kyōhan: The Master Text.* Please study Chapter 4 in that book for detailed explanations and beautiful photographs. This book, however, includes several sheets that graphically show the movements and patterns (embusen) for each form.

Learning a Kata

The first order of business in learning a kata is to learn the proper techniques and the correct pattern. Next, you must learn the rhythm using Master Funakoshi's cardinal points: expansion and contraction, light and heavy application of strength, and slow and fast movements.

Once these concepts have been realized, you must then begin to study and understand the applications and fighting techniques in the katas. Katas, therefore, can be considered forms of actual combat. You will learn from your instructor the application of the moves in each kata. Eventually, after thousands of repetitions, you can begin to develop your own understanding of a kata.

Pattern of Movement (Embusen)

Each kata has a particular pattern of movement (embusen). The correct line of movement for each kata will be shown with the diagram of movements for the kata. The techniques of any kata may vary, but they are always done within the framework of the embusen of that kata.

For the katas included in this book there are four embusens: the I-embusen, the T-embusen, the plus-minus-embusen, and the straight-line embusen, as shown next.

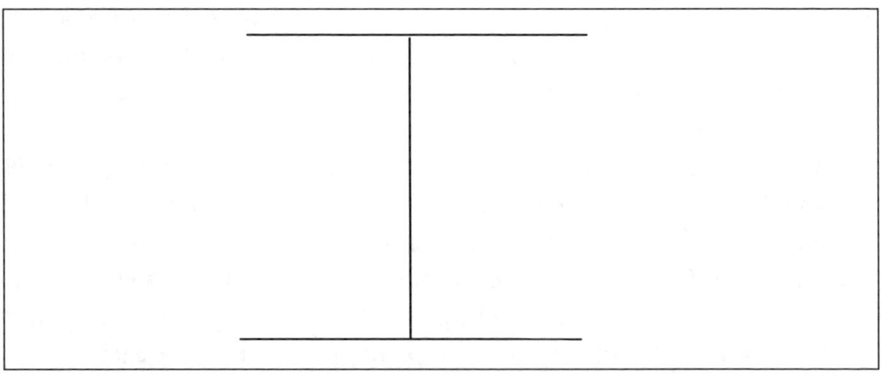

Figure 33: I-embusen used for Taikyoku Shodan, Heian Shodan, and Heian Nidan.

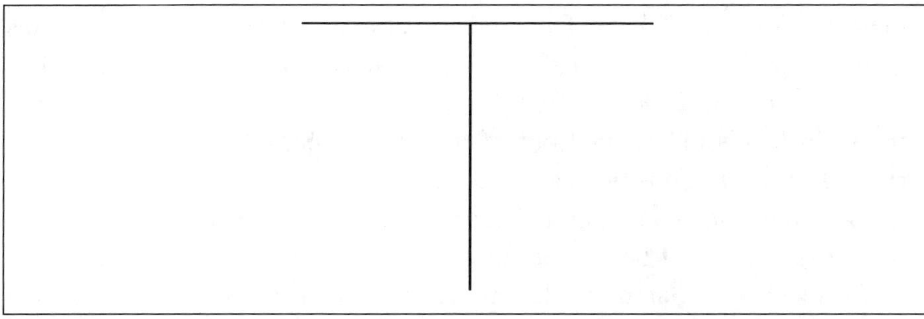

Figure 34: T-embusen used for Heian Sandan and Heian Godan.

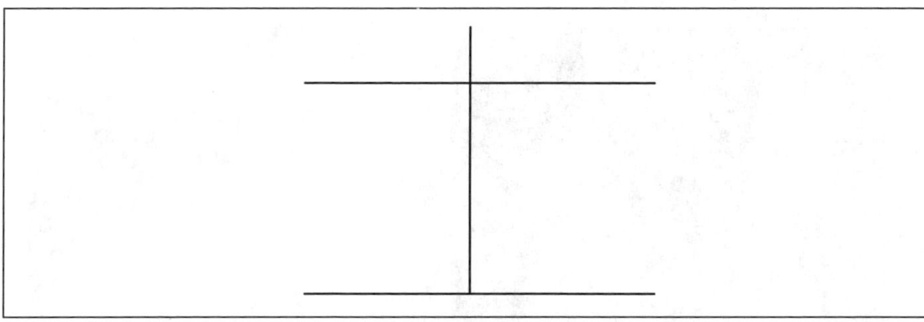

Figure 35: Plus-minus-embusen used for Heian Yodan.

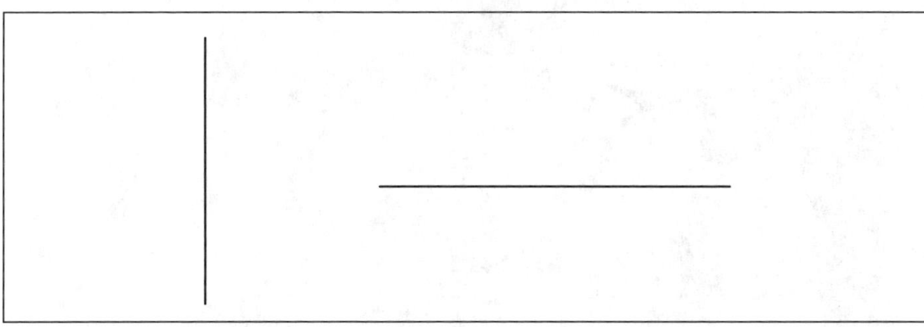

Figure 36: Two forms of the straight-line-embusen used for Ten No Kata and Tekki Shodan.

Ready Position (Yoi and Yame)

Each kata has its ready position (yoi) and its ending position (yame). The ending position can be viewed as the ending ready position. Pay close attention to these positions. Their purpose is to get you ready for the first move of the kata. The yoi and yame position for the Heian katas is the natural stance with arms and fists placed in front of the thighs. The yoi and yame position for Tekki Shodan is the feet together stance with the open hands placed in front of the groin area, left hand placed over right. The two yoi positions are shown below.

In the yoi stance breathing becomes centered in the abdomen and the mind has a sense of being able to penetrate in all directions. During our initial technique, our mind, breathing, hips, and technique move in the direction created in the kata.

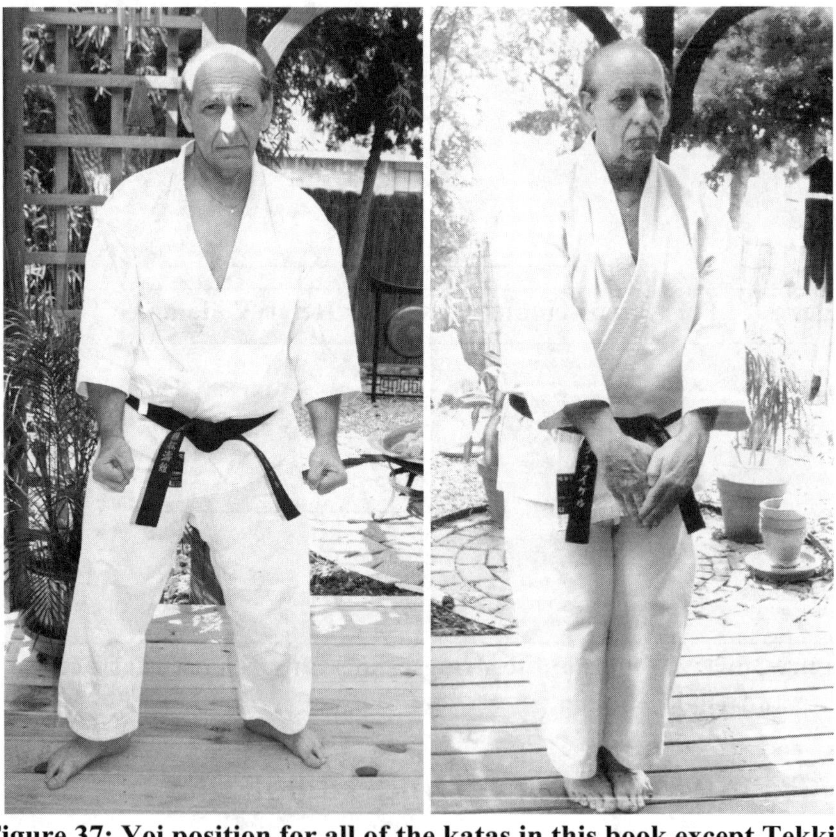

Figure 37: Yoi position for all of the katas in this book except Tekki Shodan and yoi position for Tekki Shodan.

Kiai

The kiai represent one of the strongest points in the katas. Our breathing must always be strong, but for kiais we make a noise with our exhalation to express our maximum energy. We make two kiais in each kata, usually somewhere at the middle of the form, and near its conclusion.

Kata Progression

The beginning basic katas are Taikyoku Shodan and Ten No Kata (kata of the universe). Taikyoku and Ten No Kata were introduced by Master Funakoshi several years after his public introduction of karate in Japan (1922).

Both of these katas are kihon katas. They are basic and straightforward. They both employ straight-line techniques that are found when we practice our kihon. These katas are designed to start putting our individual basic techniques into a continuous motion practice form.

After practicing Taikyoku Shodan we progress to the Heian katas. The Heian katas come from the original Pinan katas that were created by Master Anko Itosu (Master Funakoshi's teacher).

The original name for the katas, Pinan, is translated as free from harm or safe from harm. Master Funakoshi changed the name from Pinan to Heian (peaceful mind). Funakoshi stated, "Having mastered these five forms, one can be confident that he is able to defend himself competently in most situations. The meaning of the name is to be taken in this context."[5]

An interesting historical note on these Heian katas is given by Elmar T. Schmeisser, PhD, in his work entitled, *Channan: Heart of the Heians*. Dr. Schmeisser's research uncovers that Master Itosu's Pinan katas were patterned after the Chinese forms known as Chiang-Nan, later known as Channan.[6]

Legend has it that Itosu learned these katas (maybe as two long forms) from a Chinese master living in Okinawa. He is also said to have learned parts from his teacher "Bushi" Matsumura. These Channan katas were said to be derived from the southern Chinese martial art quanfa also known as gong fu in the city of Fuzhou in the Fujian Province.[7]

These facts make sense, in light of understanding how the Okinawans initially traveled and learned from their Chinese teachers in this southern city and province (see Chapter 1).

Itosu is said to have made these forms into five smaller forms, making them easier to learn. Some karate experts have also noted that Itosu incorporated movements from the more complex forms of Bassai and Kwanku into his Pinan katas.

Regardless of the historical facts, the Heian katas have a tremendous wealth of self-defense techniques that can be studied over a period of many years. The Heian katas begin to give you a sense of using your hips in many different ways with many different techniques. They have escapes, throws, vital area strikes, turning hips, dynamic in and out movements, controlling the opponent, etc. They move beyond the kihon katas and give you the feeling of continuous movement with purpose, and with more than a single option for application. The Heian katas should always be practiced with the intent of engaging an opponent. Otherwise, they become just a patterned, dance-like routine.

Taikyoku Shodan (First Cause Number One

This is the archetypal karate kata. The techniques consist of the down block (gedan-barai), front punch (oi-zuki), and front stance (zenkutsu-dachi). The yoi and yame stance are natural stance. These techniques are done within the I-embusen using a particular flow and rhythm. The graphic illustration shows the movements or individual techniques of this kata. These pictures can aid you in studying the kata.

Karate-Dō Kyōhan has excellent photos and explanations of each movement. The major points to develop when practicing this kata are learning the flow and rhythm, adjusting you breathing accordingly, and learning to move the hips dynamically forward and back, open them straight to the side, and make smooth and dynamic pivots with powerfully turning hips.

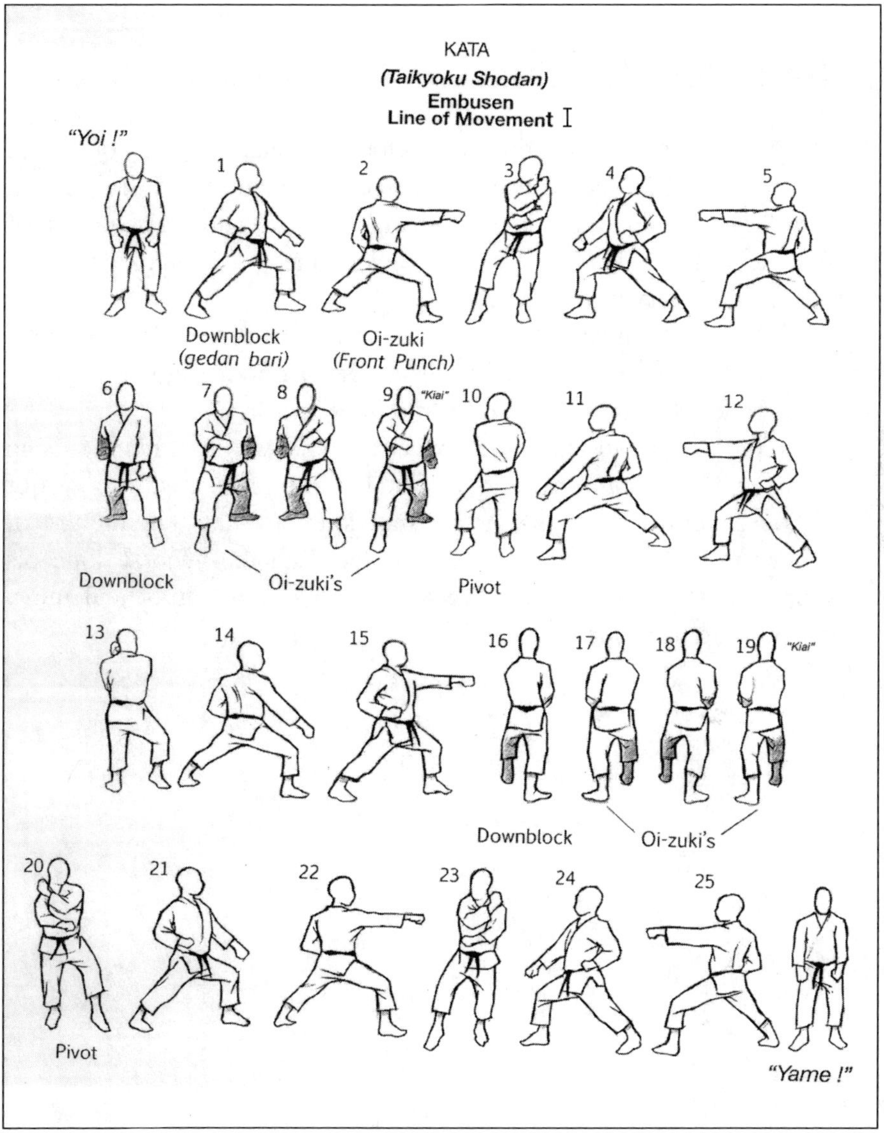
KATA
(Taikyoku Shodan)
Embusen
Line of Movement I
"Yoi !"
1
2
3
4
5
Downblock
(gedan bari)
Oi-zuki
(Front Punch)
6
7
8
9
"Kiai"
10
11
12
Downblock
Oi-zuki's
Pivot
13
14
15
16
17
18
19
"Kiai"
Downblock
Oi-zuki's
20
21
22
23
24
25
Pivot
"Yame !"

Heian Shodan (Peaceful Mind Number One)

Heian Shodan was originally taught as Heian Nidan (or Pinan Nidan). Master Funakoshi not only changed the name from the original Chinese Pinan to Heian, but he also changed its order in the sequence of the five Heian katas. He made this Heian kata the first Heian kata due to its more rudimentary movements.

This kata has many of the same basic techniques as Taikyoku Shodan. It also has the same I-embusen. Heian Shodan, however, does differ slightly in techniques, stances, and flow and rhythm.

This kata begins to teach the concept of changing rhythm, of using torite concepts (escaping techniques), and adding a back stance. Major points to develop when practicing this kata are the beginnings of understanding kata-te-dori (one-hand escape) and the general concepts that apply to torite (escaping). We also learn how to pivot and move angularly using back stance.

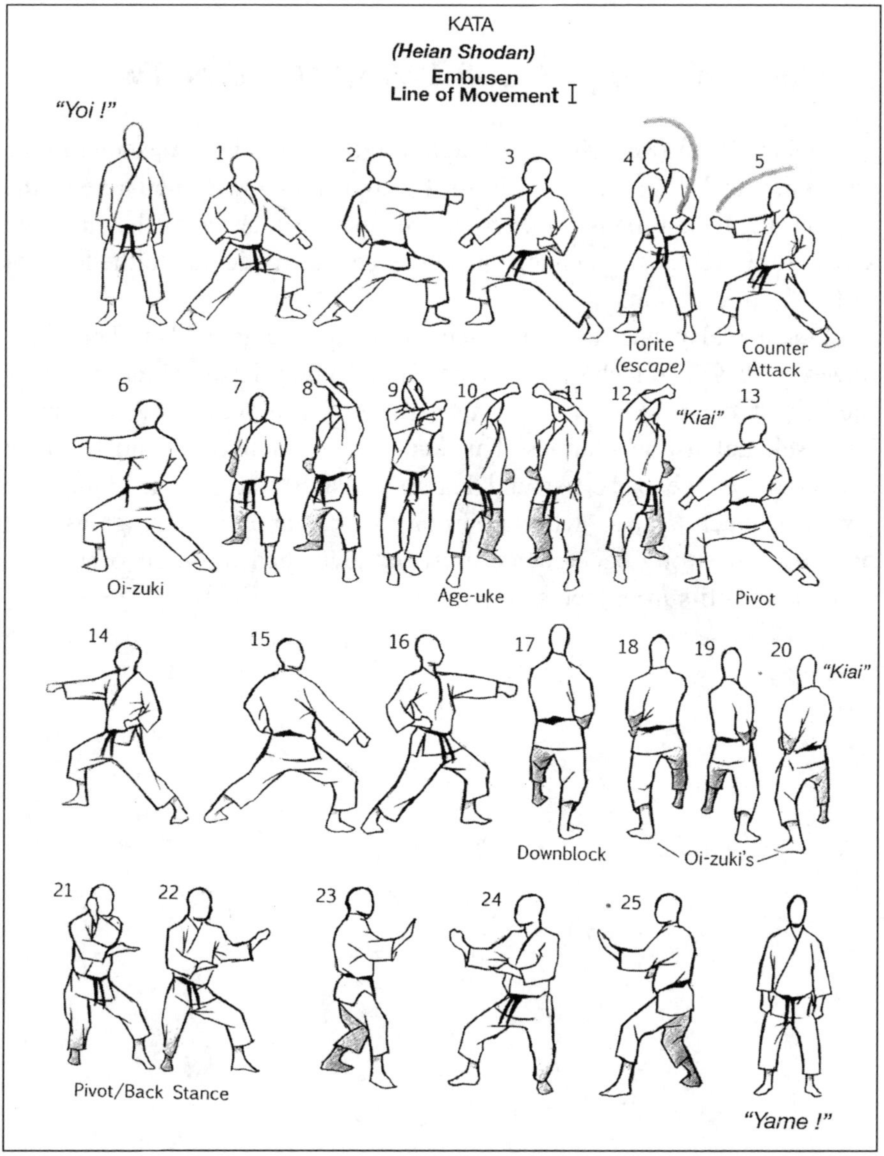
KATA
(Heian Shodan)
Embusen
Line of Movement I
"Yoi !"
1
2
3
4
5
Torite
(escape)
Counter
Attack
6
7
8
9
10
11
12
"Kiai"
13
Oi-zuki
Age-uke
Pivot
14
15
16
17
18
19
20
"Kiai"
Downblock
Oi-zuki's
21
22
23
24
25
Pivot/Back Stance
"Yame !"

Heian Nidan (Peaceful Mind Number Two)

Heian Nidan was originally taught as Heian Shodan. As stated in the discussion of Heian Shodan, Master Funakoshi changed the name of the original Chinese Pinan to Heian and reversed the order of the first two katas of this series. This change in sequence was made due to the level of difficulty of each kata.

Heian Nidan has the same I-embusen as Heian Shodan. This kata, however, differs in technique, stances, and rhythm. Heian Nidan employs the use of the back stance, the use of circular movements, and sound basic self-defense techniques. This kata also introduces the side-up kick and employs the back fist and hammer fist. Heian Nidan employs a powerful back stance with a strong back standing leg against the opponent. A strong back stance must be developed in order to begin to reap the benefits from Heian Nidan.

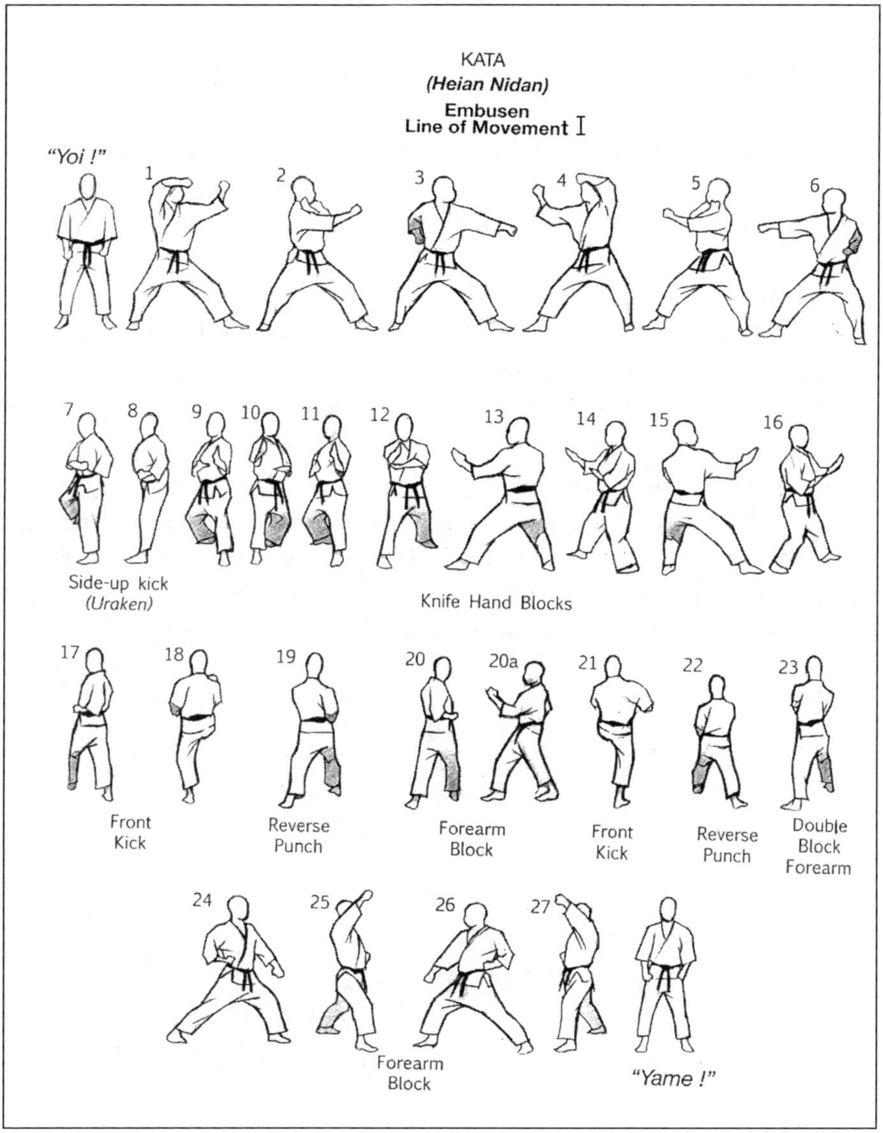
KATA
(Heian Nidan)
Embusen
Line of Movement I
"Yoi !"
1
2
3
4
5
6
7
8
9
10
11
12
13
14
15
16
Side-up kick
(Uraken)
Knife Hand Blocks
17
18
19
20
20a
21
22
23
Front Kick
Reverse Punch
Forearm Block
Front Kick
Reverse Punch
Double Block Forearm
24
25
26
27
Forearm Block
"Yame !"

Heian Sandan (Peaceful Mind Number Three)

This kata incorporates a double arm block in the beginning of the kata — a gedan-barai and ude-uke. It also lets you practice making kime as the legs come together. This kata has a T-embusen form, which differs from the previous katas.

Ohshima Sensei in his *Notes on Training* states that Heian Sandan combines both the Shōrin and Shōkei schools. He states that this kata has a much stronger Shōkei influence than the other Heian katas.[8]

This Heian kata has a lot of turning-hip movements. It has a turning torite (escaping technique) and employs the use of the kiba-dachi (horse riding stance). There are many good techniques for realistic in-close fighting (the use of back fist and stamps). Because of the turning and spinning nature of some of the moves, you will learn how to have a solid, balanced center of gravity. We also get a sense of using our elbows and using the legs and knees to protect our centerline (vital areas).

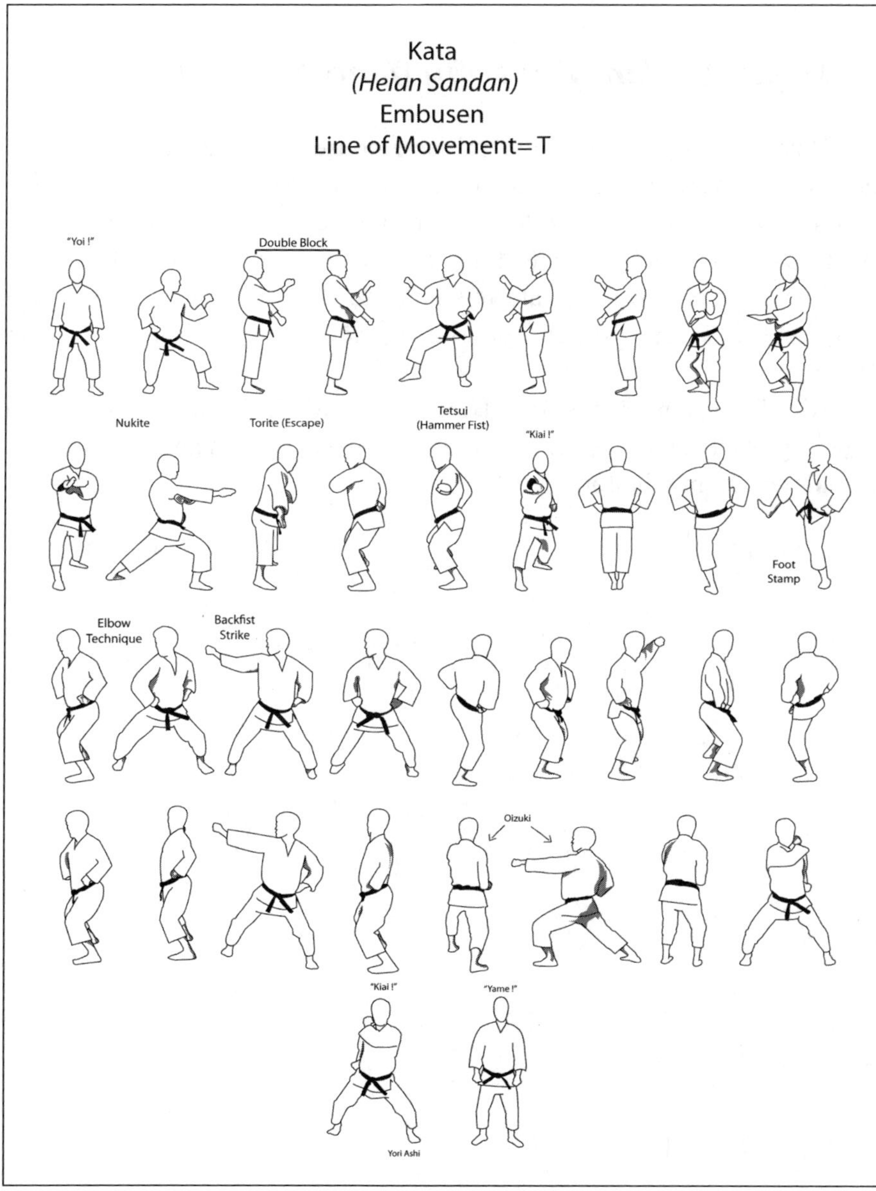
Kata
(Heian Sandan)
Embusen
Line of Movement= T
"Yoi !"
Double Block
Nukite
Torite (Escape)
Tetsui
(Hammer Fist)
"Kiai !"
Foot
Stamp
Elbow
Technique
Backfist
Strike
Oizuki
"Kiai !"
"Yame !"
Yori Ashi

Heian Yodan (Peaceful Mind Number Four)

Heian Yodan uses the plus-minus-embusen. This kata employs the use of open hand blocks and attacks. It also employs the back fist strike and has a variety of self-defense techniques including kakiwake (a realistic opening and escape technique) and a powerful knee strike.

The beginning of this kata is similar to that of Heian Nidan except that the hands are open as opposed to the closed fist form in Heian Nidan.

All of the Heian katas from Heian Nidan to Heian Godan begin with a strong back stance. They also employ the back stance in various techniques during the form.

KATA
(Heian Yodan)
Embusen
Line of Movement = ±

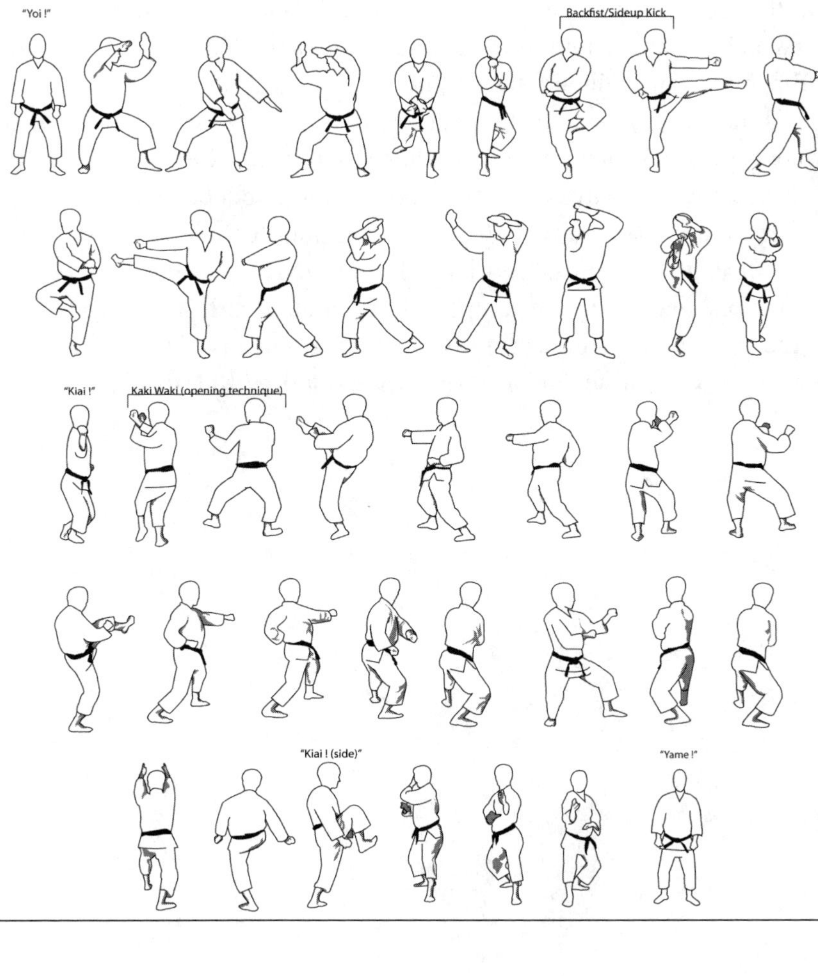

Heian Godan (Peaceful Mind Number Five)

Heian Godan is the fifth and last kata in the Heian series. This kata has the same T-embusen as Heian Sandan. This kata illustrates Master Funakoshi's cardinal points of practicing a kata: slow and fast, expansion and contraction, light and heavy power.

Some might consider this kata as being the most difficult and most athletic of the Heian series. This kata will really begin to develop the skill necessary to advance to the more senior, independent katas. Heian Godan is the first kata that employs a jumping technique, which helps to develop your balance as you land. Heian Godan introduces several new techniques (including the jump), a heaven and earth throwing technique at the end, and an uppercut fist to the opponent's jaw. Heian Godan employs six of the seven basic stances (excluding fudō-dachi).

KATA

(Heian Godan)

Embusen

Line of Movement = T

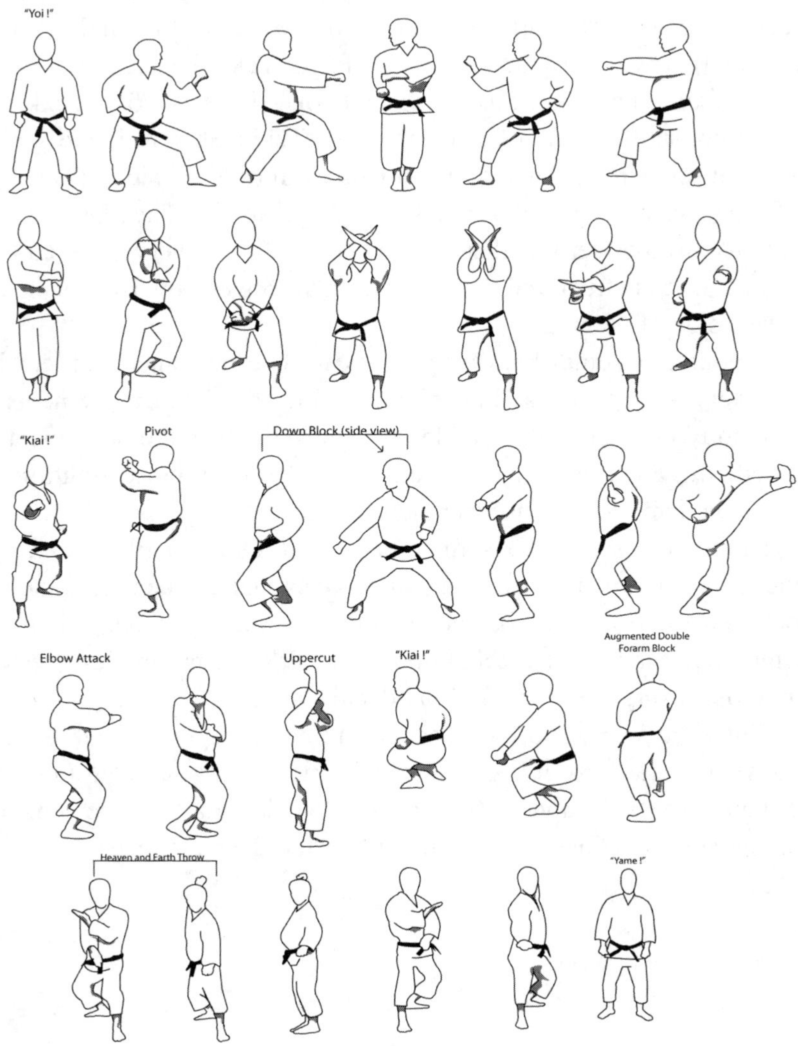

Tekki Shodan (Armed Warrior Riding Horse Number One)

Ohshima Sensei translates the meaning of Tekki to "Armed Warrior Riding Horse." This kata was originally practiced by Master Funakoshi under the name of Naifanchi (inner battle or in the middle of the battlefield). There are actually three different Tekki katas: Tekki Shodan, Tekki Nidan, and Tekki Sandan. This book covers the first Tekki kata, Tekki Shodan. The line of movement for Tekki Shodan is the straight-line-embusen with a lateral movement from side to side. The kata is performed using the kiba-dachi stance exclusively. The yoi and yame positions are the feet-together stance. This kata is a very short and very exact kata. It is structured to have identical movements (mirror images) for each side of the body.

This kata is somewhat of a paradox in that the stance and legs have to be very strong and solidly planted while the hand movements and upper body must be soft, flexible, and relaxed. Once the movements are learned, this kata should be practiced for good in-close fighting with many excellent self-defense techniques.

There are back-fists, some very good elbow strikes, and close punches. There are also returning wave kicks that can be used to not only block, but to destroy the balance of the opponent by kicking their outer or inner leg. Many of the techniques in the Tekki katas are designed to be very close, using the powerful kiba-dachi stance.

This kata is very short and seems simple. The opposite is true. This is an advanced kata that a beginner can learn. When you begin to practice this kata, you will soon understand that it takes many more repetitions than the Heians before you start to understand the techniques.

KATA
(Tekki Shodan)
Embusen
Line of Movement = ——

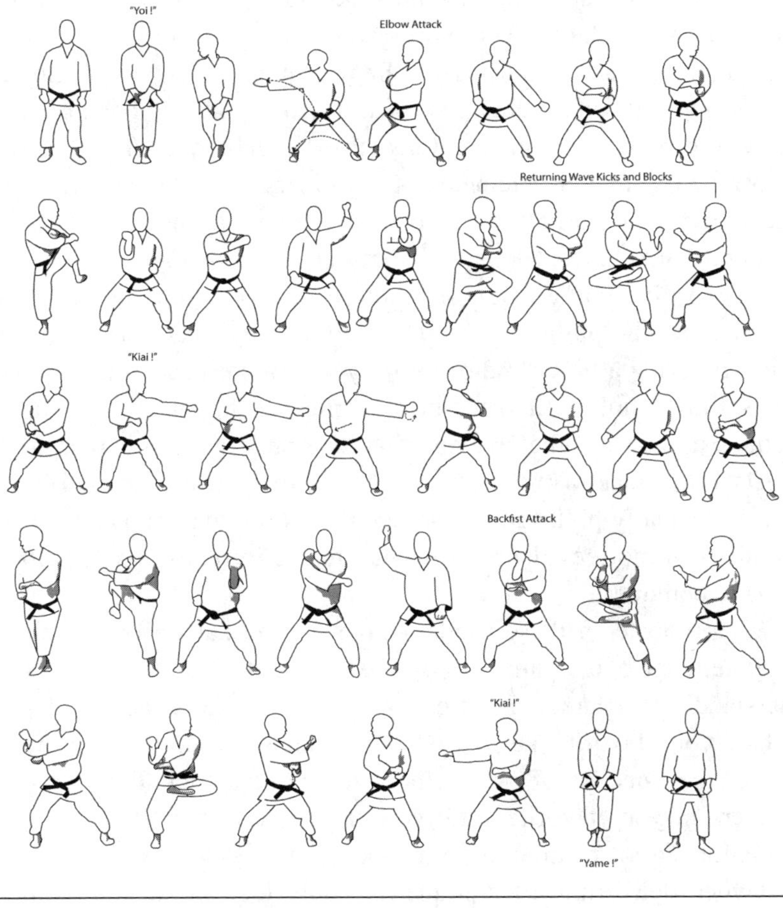

Summary of Kata Practice

I quoted Ohshima Sensei at the beginning of this chapter saying that "katas hold crystals of knowledge which are passed down from senior to junior."[9] This statement especially holds true when it comes to understanding the many applications that exist within each kata. There can be several different interpretations of applications in the various kata movements. There are the basic and there are also the hidden or implied applications.

The various applications become clearer as you repeat the movements in the katas. The more each kata is practiced, the more you begin to understand the purpose of the movements. As you progress, you will develop a favorite kata and repeat it many times. Polishing one kata will help to polish all katas, and actually all techniques. In other words, the core fundamental elements are universal and create a type of systematic infusion into the subconscious mind and body of the trainee. At around 5,000 times, a kata will start to be your own.

Let me give you a prime example of a technique you can study in kata practice: the pulling hand. The pulling hand that comes to the hip while delivering a block and becomes your counterattack often translates to unsettling, pulling-in, or unbalancing an opponent. In my own practice, it has become evident that not only does my pulling hand connect both sides of my body, but that a realistically applied block or parry will usually pull, turn, or somehow disrupt the opponent. This will become even more evident when you engage in realistic self-defense or combat techniques.

When you learn these fundamentals in one kata, the core elements will "network-over" and apply to all katas and to an overall understanding of karate practice. When you make a powerful pulling hand in your favorite kata, you can make it in all katas. When you develop the concept of your elbow, underarm, back foot, or relaxed shoulders in your favorite kata, you can make this in all katas and, by association, in all techniques. Katas also show you how the body must relax when delivering a technique and only focusing at the moment of impact.

For combat, the movements in katas should be studied with the mindset of defending yourself using these dynamic techniques. The movements in katas, especially in the five Heians, hold hidden a wealth of combat techniques that should be reviewed, studied, and practiced by all serious students.

You should also remember that when these forms were created, most experts had a real working knowledge of throwing techniques, pressure points, and vital areas. They also had an understanding of stick fighting and using other weapons. These katas, therefore, include many self-defense techniques similar to modern grappling and boxing, as well as traditional karate techniques that are taught in many schools today. Try to understand how your technique can unbalance and eventually incapacitate your opponent. The applications (bunkai) should give you a sense of following-up with an alternative move or technique. This is not always overt, but many times implied.

Hopefully, your instructor will shed some light on the meaning of the movements and the mentality necessary when applying them. These two concepts are extremely important if karate students expect to advance their understanding of the art. Otherwise, katas will just remain a string of patterned movements that resemble some type of dance routine.

Always practice your forms with the mindset of engaging an opponent. When you begin to practice your favorite kata, ask the question, "How would I use this (or something similar) in actual combat?" Make a practical application in kumite practice especially during one-time or three-time sparring. Your katas will then have a realistic foundation and will help to give life to your understanding of the applications. Never just look at katas as simply a patterned movement, but look at katas as a tool for your combat ability.

Suggested reading

Karate-Dō Kyōhan by Gichin Funakoshi, Translated by Tsutomu Ohshima. Chapter 4. The Kata, pp. 34-208.

---

[1] Tsutomu Ohshima, *Notes on Training*, pp. 5-7.
[2] Gichin Funakoshi, *Karate-Dō Kyōhan*, p. 41.
[3] *Ibid.*, p. 40.
[4] *Ibid.*, p. 8.
[5] *Ibid.*, p. 35.
[6] Elmar Schmeisser, *Channan*, p. 2
[7] *Ibid.*, p. 2
[8] Tsutomu Ohshima, *Notes on Training*, p. 20.
[9] Tsutomu Ohshima, *Notes on Training*, pp. 5-7.

7. Basic Sparring (Kumite)

"Looking through the enemy's eyes," actually means looking at our own weaknesses and weak moments, as well as at others. As martial artists we must always see ourselves as the enemy does in order to prepare realistically.... Don't lock into the structure of the method of practice, but search for what it is trying to teach you... always think of training for situations of no rules...[1]

Don DePree
Shotokan Karate of America

Basic sparring is sometimes referred to as prearranged sparring practice. In this practice we specify who will attack and who will defend, and also what type of attack will be delivered and to what general area of the body.

Even though basic sparring is prearranged, the quote at the beginning of the chapter from Don DePree is the essence of our kumite practice. Mr. DePree was one of the top senior instructors under Ohshima Sensei in Shotokan Karate of America. Mr. DePree's combat ability and expertise in kumite was of the highest caliber. What he said is that our practice must be realistic, applicable, and honest. It is not just some systemized way of going through the motions.

Keeping this thought in mind, let us review some basic concepts of our sparring and then look at the practices that allow us to put our instruction into practical application. The first type of sparring is basic

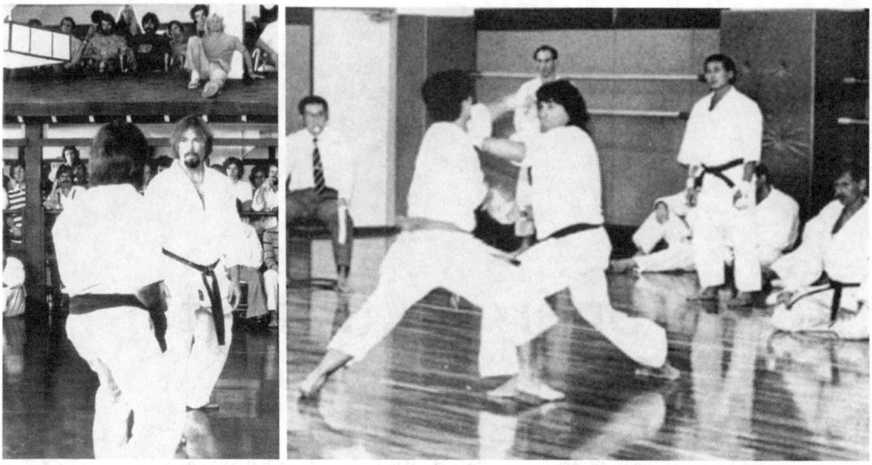

Figure 38: Don DePree facing Tom Muzila. Tom Muzila engages an opponent.

one-time sparring with a fist attack. This practice can be later expanded to three-time sparring, kicking matches (using kicks for offense and defense or both), and free sparring practice.

Basic Concepts

Distance and Other Elements (Ma)

The initial concept of ma seems to be distance but the true translation of the term ma involves timing, mentality, ranking, and rhythm. Ohshima Sensei in *Notes on Training* talks about the five stages of learning about ma describing what he calls the alpha, which includes the nature of the opponent, size, strength, tendencies, etc.[2] The more complicated components of ma will be your concern when you become more experienced senior students. This understanding is a natural and organic development for senior students who practice for many years and have a realistic sense of an opponent.

For beginners, we start with a very basic understanding of ma. The basic concept is simply the distance between two opponents. If we are too close, we are inside the ma and cannot escape from a good opponent.

Too far is also unrealistic because we are not in danger and will never get a sense of actual combat.

We must practice finding the proper ma in relation to our opponent. Ma is not something that can be intellectualized or talked about. It must be practiced and experienced with your classmates.

We begin to experience this distance with a drill that helps set the proper distance. We should always remember several things in relation to setting ma: there is only one ma between opponents, karate has the longest ma of the weaponless martial arts, and ma must be developed into something that is sensed.

These concepts should be understood as we begin to learn about ma by extending our arms to reach each other and then moving slightly back. In "real life" we don't go around touching people to set our distance. Again we should understand the concept which this exercise is teaching. Animals, especially if they are feral, have a real understanding of ma. Human beings also have that understanding, but it has become hidden in our subconscious because we don't practice using it or because we don't understand the signs that our subconscious mind gives us.

Felines are predators and usually have good combat ability. Cats usually attack with their jaws and swipe and grab with their sharp claws. That being said, cats have an intuitive sense of ma. Once they decide to attack, their powerful hind legs and hips move their jaws and grabbing claws at their opponents. We can really get a good sense of ma by studying cats (large or small).

Eyes

Looking into the opponent's eyes very strongly demonstrates your focused and courageous mind. Practice looking at your opponent without blinking, looking down, or looking away. Ohshima Sensei in *Notes on Training* says, "The eyes are the windows of the mind …, the actions of your eyes show your mentality."[3]

Fighting Spirit

"What is the most important element that can help a warrior survive in combat or battle? Spirit! A true warrior must have fearless spirit

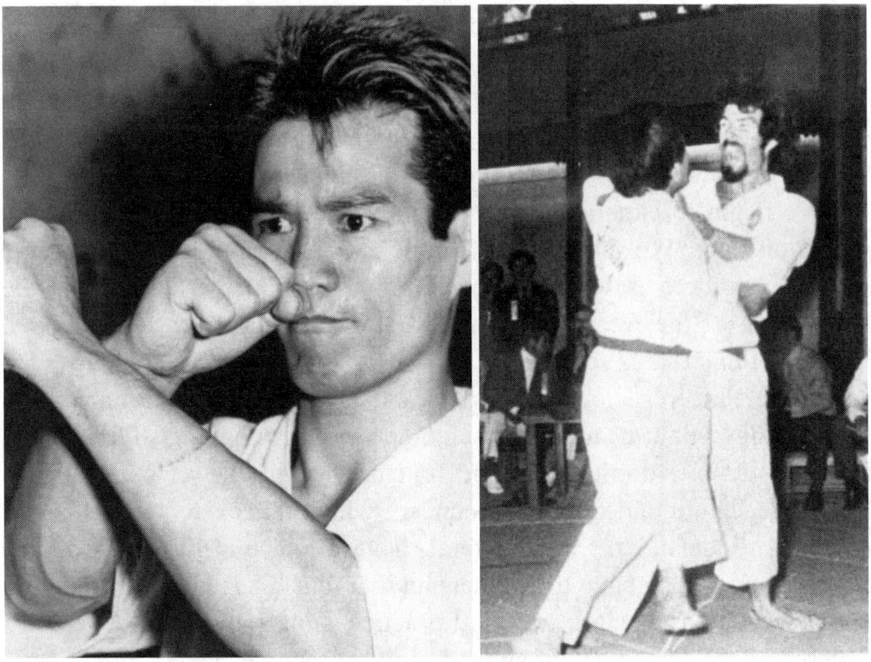

Figure 39: Ohshima Sensei displays his powerful eyes. Don DePree demonstrates his fighting spirit.

against all odds. It doesn't mean he doesn't fear anything, but he knows how to control and redirect fear to be more effective in surviving and dominating his opponent."[4]

This fighting spirit is sometimes referred to as fudōshin which translates to indomitable spirit or warrior heart. This is a mental edge. Confidence, positive mind, and positive outlook give a person an advantage. This concept should not be taken lightly. It will serve you well to develop a strong fighting spirit. This can be done by hard and dedicated training sessions (especially like those conducted at SKA's Special Trainings), making strong kiais, and always looking strongly into your opponents eyes. Again this is experiential, not a topic for a discussion in a classroom.

Basic Sparring Practice Drill

This practice will consist of the block and counterattack portion of Ten No Kata (Kata of Heaven). The basic blocks are employed to block an offensive technique and dynamically apply a counterattack. Master Funakoshi devoted an entire book to the techniques of Ten No Kata entitled *Karate-Dō Nyūmon*.

The parts of Ten No Kata described here are combinations using the five blocks described in the basics section followed by a striking technique. The counterattack is usually a reverse punch.

This block-punch combination will first be developed when we practice basics. As we move beyond making our basic blocks to the side and then moving forward, we eventually step back with blocks in a more realistic fashion. We then add counterattacks to the blocks, making two techniques with one feeling.

When we start doing kumite in practice, we start by lining up directly across from an opponent with both sides in a natural stance. At the command, both sides will practice the same Ten No Kata form and then return to the natural stance. This can be done with all six combination techniques. See the illustrations for these techniques.

The next phase of sparring practice has one side standing in a front stance in a down block position. For example, left leg forward, left arm in a down block position (parallel to the left thigh), right arm and fist in a pulling hand at the right hip. This stance is made as a preparatory stance for delivering a front punch. The opposite side will stand in a natural stance and perform the Ten No Kata block/counterattack technique that was practiced by both sides in the previous exercise.

As we go through all of the techniques, one side will attack and the other side will block and counterattack. The area of the attack will be pre-arranged, either middle level (chūdan) or upper level (jōdan). The person who is defending will be using a defensive technique appropriate for the area being attacked. These blocks will be followed with a counterattack.

The initial distance for this drill will be pretty wide (outside of ma). You will be moving at the same time with a command. Eventually, the distance between opponents becomes narrower. The drill is then done without counting. Finally, the practice changes to one-time sparring with counting and then without counting.

Basic Fist and Open Hand Blocks and Counterattacks

1.All techniques begin in natural stance.

2.(Step back) downblock (gedanbarai)

3. Reverse punch (gyakuzuki)

4. Inside forearm block (ude uke)

5. Reverse punch

6. Knife hand block (shuto uke)

7. Spearhand (nukite)

8. Hammer block (tetsui uke)

9. Reverse punch

10. Rising block (age uke)

11. Reverse punch (gyakuzuki)

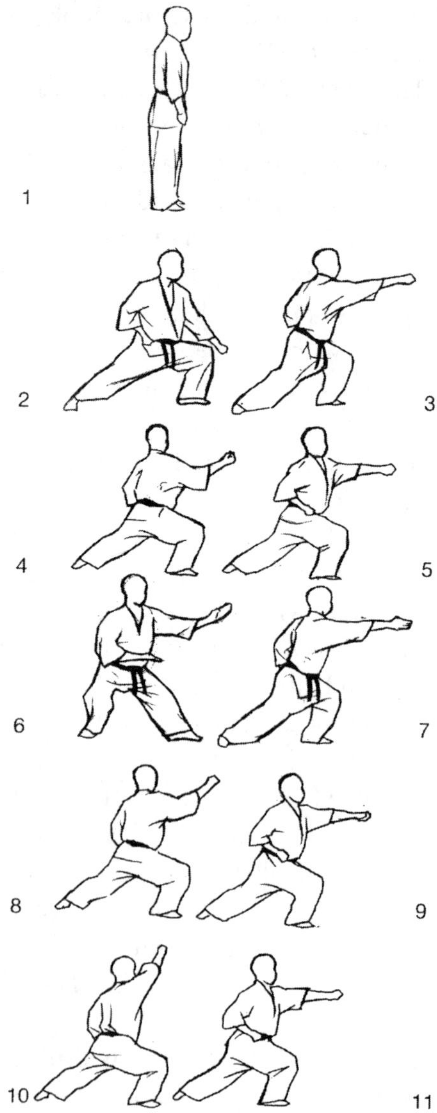

Basic One-Time Sparring (Kihon Ippon Gumite

There are three major elements to basic one-time sparring. The attacker makes an attack trying to hit a specified target with a specified technique. The defender blocks the attack. Immediately following the block, the defender makes an effective counterattack, which is controlled. Each of these elements is described below.

This form of kumite as well as all other forms begin and end with rei (bow). This signifies that we will respect our opponent and give them our best effort whether it is offensive or defensive. Both sides will learn only if each side is giving their strong, honest feeling.

I hope that you realize this and give this portion of practice your best effort. You will never experience what it is like to be attacked or deliver a powerful attack unless you commit yourself in practice. Remember we learn and gain insight as we interact with each other.

When we are first learning this practice, the attacking side will set the distance by extending their arms and stepping back, just to the edge of ma. Basic one-time sparring is done by having both sides stand outside of the ma. The attacking side takes one step forward into the preparatory stance (front stance, down block position) at the exact ma for this combination of opponents.

Attacking

Attacking in one-time sparring is customarily made with a front punch from a down block position with front stance. The attacking side sets the distance and assumes the ready stance described above. The area of attack is designated by the leader prior to the engagement, either middle level (solar plexus) or upper level (face area). Attack by making your strongest front punch* to the designated area. Watch your opponent's eyes and punch through the target making a strong back leg

---

* Seniors attacking juniors make a front punch that is appropriate for the junior's level.

connection as you complete the movement. (See the section on hand techniques in Chapter 4 and comments by Jim Sagawa.)

Basic Ippon Kumite

(One Time Engagement Match)

Attacker; preparatory stance, downblock position in a front stance.

Defender; natural stance in preparation for an attack. Fists in front of thighs.

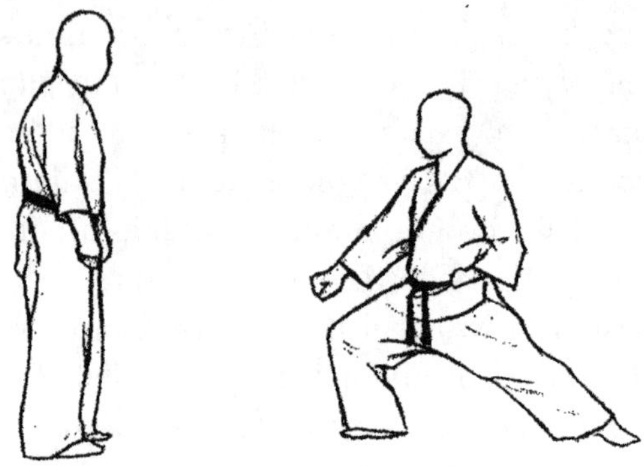

1

Attacker; attacks with middle Level oizuki (front punch).

Defender; steps back and applies gedan barai (down block).

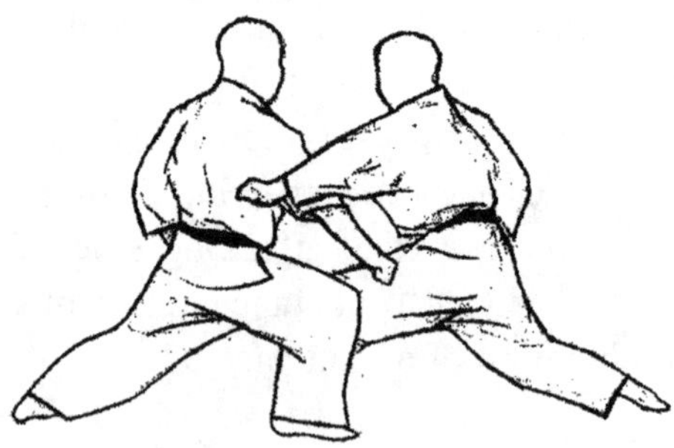

2

Defender; completes defense With gyakuzi (reverse punch / counter punch).

3

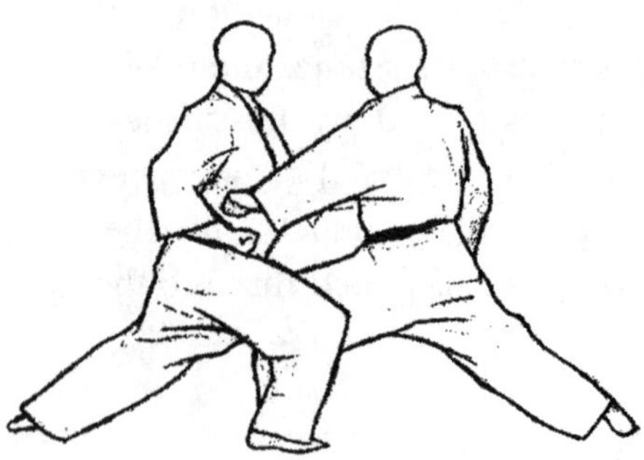

Blocking Concepts and Counterattacking

Blocking an offensive technique should stop the attack from striking you, and it can also disrupt the rhythm of the attacker or unsettle or unbalance them. Any of these can create an opening for a counterattack. Both the block and counterattack should be made with one breath; two techniques are made with one feeling.

The blocking techniques should be executed using the core foundational values discussed in Chapter 3: a strong standing leg, a good pulling hand, and the elbow in close to the body with little or no power in the shoulders. The technique should be combined with a strong outward breath emanating from your lower abdomen area.

At this stage, your standing leg is very important. That is why when we begin to practice Ten No Kata we stand in a front stance with a very strong back leg. This back leg connection will ensure that both sides of the body are connected to a powerful and dynamic hip. When the hip is connected, the defender is able to easily deflect the attack and also able to unsettle the balance of the attacker. (See the illustrations.)

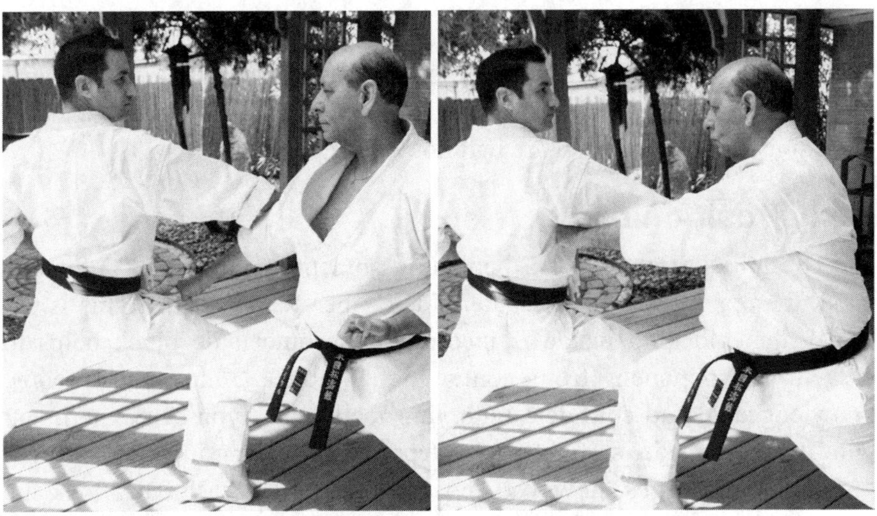

Figure 40: Attacker — oi-zuki (front punch middle level), Defender — gedan-barai (down block) gyaku-zuki (reverse punch middle level).

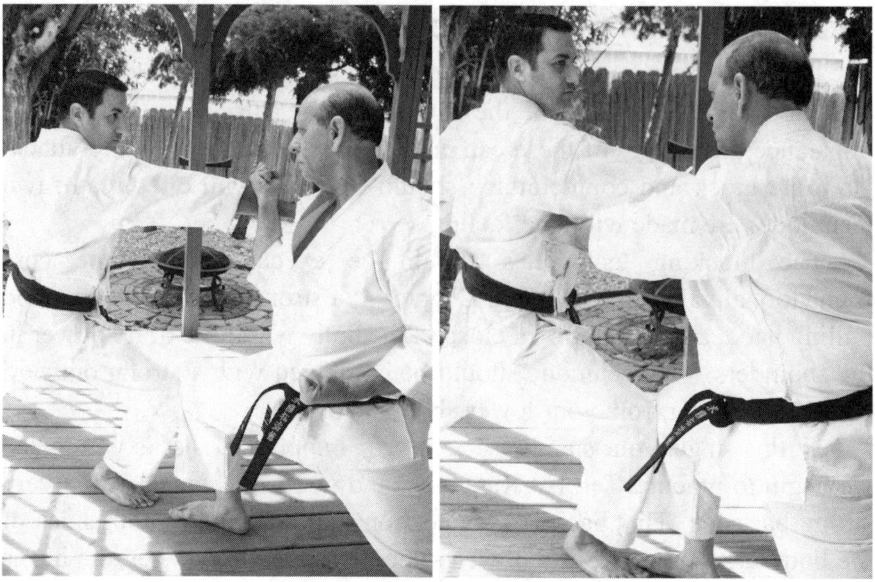

Figure 41: Attacker — oi-zuki (front punch middle level), Defender — ude-uke (inside forearm block middle level) gyaku-zuki (reverse punch middle level).

The counterattack that follows can initially be delivered in the form of a reverse punch. This should be done almost instantly with the same breath after the opponent is blocked. The defender must learn to execute this counterattack to a vital area without hesitation.

Body Positioning

The initial strategy for a beginning student should be to defend or block the opponent from the outer side of the attacking arm. This is not to say that blocking inside is incorrect. The outer side block helps to prevent the opponent from continuing to attack. Once you become knowledgeable and confident with your techniques, you can experiment with outside, inside, straight back, stepping in, turning hips, etc. During the beginning stages, however, most people find it easier to block the attack by stepping back on an angle. This moves the body to an advantageous position with the hips out of the line of attack.

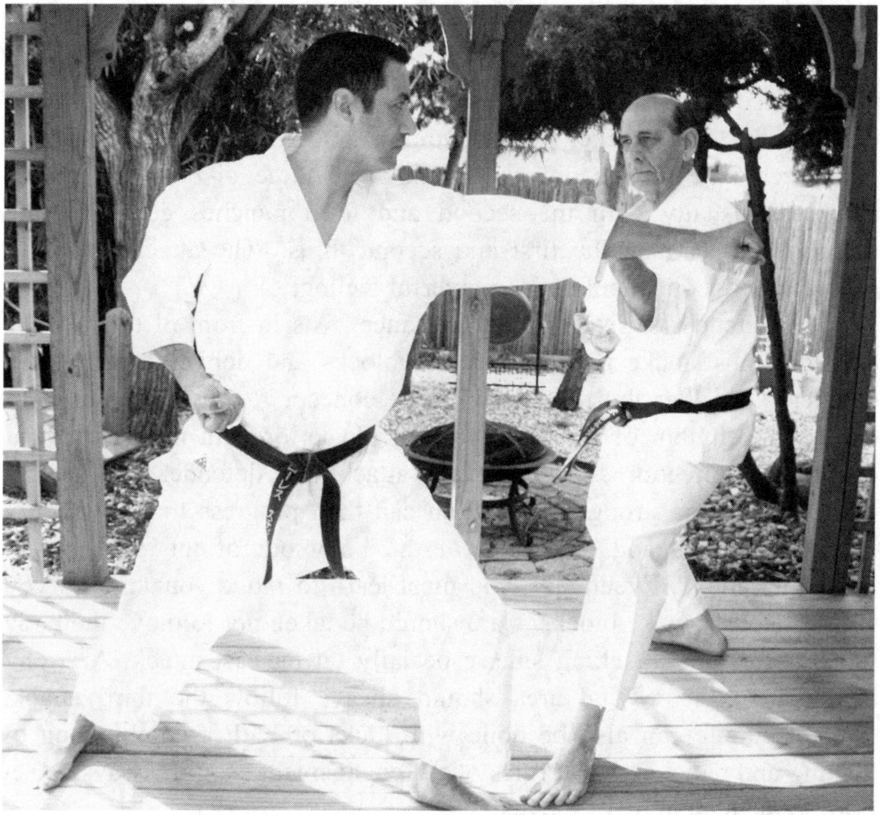

Figure 42: Basic one-time sparring, angled block with shutō-uke.

Through trial and error you will find that it becomes more difficult to block a powerful attack if the hips are not connected to the standing leg or if the hips are left behind, creating a square feeling against the opponent with the centerline and vital areas exposed.

Three-Time Sparring (Sanbon Gumite)

In three-time sparring the attacker makes three successive attacks to a designated area with a designated technique. The defender blocks or escapes from the three attacks and makes an effective counterattack, which is controlled. This form of sparring should be developed after you have practiced basic one-time sparring.

The match begins with rei. The attacker stands at the closest safe distance (ma) and steps backward into a front stance. The attacker then makes three successive attacks (usually oi-zuki) to the designated area of the defender. The attacker should avoid making a reverse punch or some other technique that is not an oi-zuki. The three oi-zukis should be complete, usually with the second and third punches coming more closely together than the first and second thrust. The attacker tries to overwhelm the opponent with a powerful feeling.

The defender starts in a natural stance, fists in front of thighs. The defender must make three successive blocks and deliver a successful counterattack after the third attack. The concept for the defender is to disrupt the rhythm of the attacker with blocks or with movement that changes the direction and flow of the attack. The defender can initially work on making strong blocks. You can then progress to dynamically moving the hips and centerline of the body out of the path of the oncoming attack. Eventually, you must learn to move your hips as you simultaneously make blocks. Care should be taken not to move the body too far from the attacking side, especially on the last attack. A strong counterattack to a vital area should always follow the third attack. Sanbon gumite can also be done with kicks or with a combination of kicking and punching. The rules of the engagement should always be set prior to the beginning of the match.

Three-time attack should not turn into a brawl or free for all. Care must be taken that both sides understand the parameters of this form of kumite. When done properly, sanbon gumite is an excellent form of sparring and will really help to form a strong mind and give you a sense of moving and reacting to a strong opponent.

Chudan (Middle Level)

Sanbon Gumite
Three-Time Engagement Match

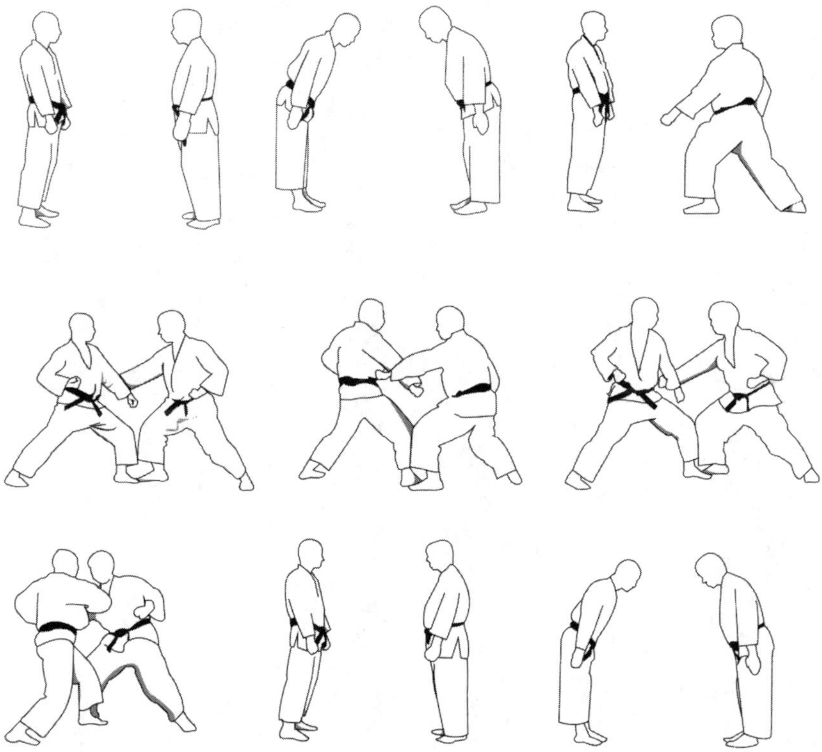

Jodan (Upper Level)

Sanbon Gumite

Three-time engagement match

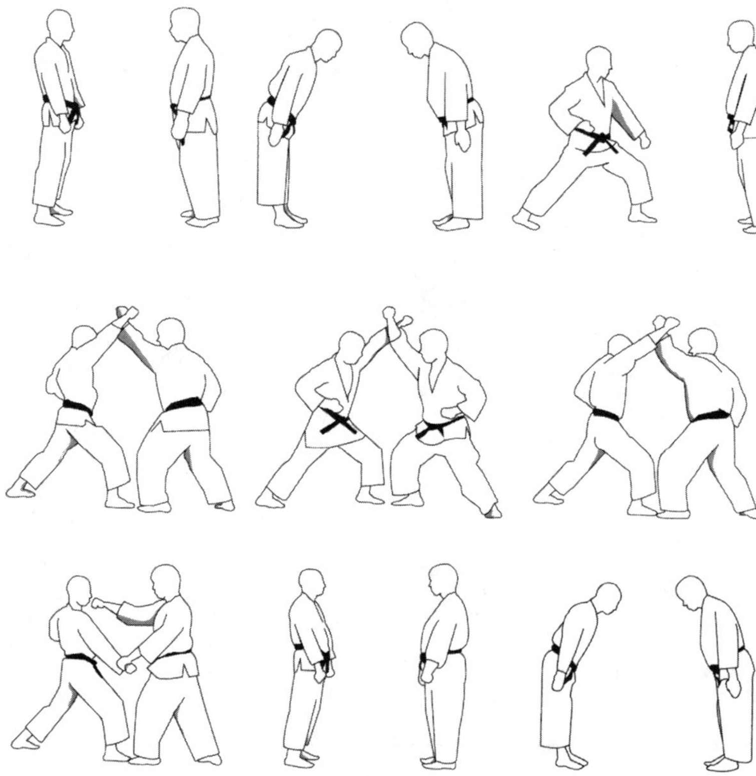

Summary

The basic one-time sparring and three-time sparring should not be viewed as only a systemized form of engagement. There are real lessons to be learned. Begin to understand how our practice is interrelated.

For instance, a defender standing squarely against an attacker opens the entire centerline. But what is this teaching us? Maybe it shows that we need to be able to move in such a way that we are able to protect our vulnerable areas. Real situations may force us to defend from very vulnerable or open positions. We need to practice moving quickly and judiciously.

The concept of ma is extremely important. So is looking into your opponents' eyes to understand their feelings and noting their breathing patterns. Physical confrontations usually begin with a verbal disagreement that escalates to shouting, threats, pushing, grappling, etc. (Of course, this is not true in all situations.) Basic kumite practice can begin to teach you to avoid a situation or, if necessary, defend yourself with confidence and purpose.

Finally, young people can become very passionate about their feelings and can sometimes let their emotions dictate their actions. I hope that by practicing karate-dō, you will come to realize that the most difficult opponent you will face in life is the "ugly part" that exists in yourself.

Hopefully, our practice can begin to help us to face this opponent and to eventually overcome it. The more we practice, the more we polish our character. That's why our practice of karate-dō spans our lifetimes.

Suggested Reading

Karate-Dō Kyōhan by Gichin Funakoshi, translated by Tsutomu Ohshima. Chapter 4. The Kata, pp. 202-208 (Ten No Kata Omote), Chapter 5. Engagement Matches, pp. 211-223.

---

[1] Don DePree, Shotokan Karate of America: *Relevance of Karate Practice.*
[2] Tsutomu Ohshima, *Notes on Training*, p. 218.
[3] Tsutomu Ohshima, *Notes on Training*, p. 212.
[4] Tom Muzila, *Mental Karate*, p. 137.

8. Conclusion

> Fulfilling one's potential, both physically and mentally, is a continuing, lifelong process dependent largely upon being motivated to a lifetime of training, by an activity that stimulates self-perfection. (Karate can be such an activity.)... So, over the years it has been found that as the original self-defense need for Karate training grew less and less, the only factor which would motivate one to a lifetime of training, which would then allow one to reach his full potential both physically and mentally, was to use Karate for that reason (to perfect oneself).[1]
>
> *Don DePree*
> *Shotokan Karate of America*

All of the Ways to self-improvement are said to contain two distinct wings: the technical aspect of training and transcendence of technique.[2] A person who continually trains in these wings will begin to manifest a certain purity of spirit as they polish themselves as human beings. Karate-dō is a path that can help a person work toward this ideal.

The traditional Ways, including karate-dō, are technically difficult and take many years of dedicated practice for any meaningful development. I think it is safe to say that traditional karate practice helps us to attain certain positive attributes: physical conditioning, combat ability, self-confidence, leadership qualities, friendship, plus an overall sense of well being. However, as one advances in life one realizes that the sport aspect of karate is not where the dō or Way has its roots. Reiterating the thoughts of Mr. DePree at the beginning of this chapter, our karate practice is a practice to master the self. To understand that means our everyday life becomes our contest, in essence it becomes our opponent.

Students often ask how long they should continue to practice to be good or to become an expert. They also ask what black belt degree I have.

The answer to the first question is simple. If you are a serious student of karate, you should practice until you die. The answer to the second question is also simple. I give my rank and explain that it is a lifelong process of self-discovery, not of yesterday or tomorrow, but of the present and of a lifetime. We live in a microwave "quick-gratification" society. We want to receive instant knowledge that will allow us to present ourselves as some type of expert. We must realize that there is no "microwave" karate. Real advancement will only come with steady, disciplined, hard practice. This can become boring to someone who wants instant success.

Practicing a Way creates a path to polish and develop yourself as a productive and positive human being, someone who enhances society in a meaningful way.

Karate-dō is not a religion nor is it a cultist system of dogmatic beliefs. On the contrary, karate-dō can truly help you to excel in whatever endeavor you choose: being the best student you can be, a valued employee, a leader of your chosen field, a meaningful religious minister of your chosen faith, a devoted family member (husband, wife, parent, etc.).

Karate-dō, as a martial art, goes beyond its sports association. This book is designed to introduce the beginning student to the martial arts. Hopefully, it will help you explore, through the direct experience of practicing, the relationship between ethics, philosophy, and the rigors of strenuous practice. It is designed specifically to challenge you and give you a wake-up call that pushes you out of a sleepwalk through life.

We must begin to wake up to our true nature and our potential in life. "If a jewel is not polished, it will not shine. Even a diamond with all of its brilliance will not shine until it is polished."[3] Human beings are no different. Our shiny natures will only shine if they are polished. Martial arts provide one path human beings can follow to achieve their true natures.

However, one should never become so closed-minded or dogmatic about their style of practice that they fail to grasp the concepts of what their art is teaching. On a larger scale, you must also embrace the real meaning of dō in karate-dō.

The techniques of fighting differ from martial art to martial art, but the waza, ki, and shin (technique, spirit energy, and attitude) must form one single whole. This is imperative for what the Zen masters would call "right action."[4] Without these ingredients, there can be no right action. If this right action is not present, we then become like predators that are strong with an instinctive desire to always win or dominate. Predators can't go beyond their own selfish egos. We, as humans, must rise above these feelings. We are not wild animals.[5]

There is a story told by a disciple of the great Lao Tsu about a king who wanted to own a champion fighting cock.[6]

> He arranged for one of his subjects to train a champion cock for him. So the man began training this particular rooster in all of the combat techniques to be a champion. The king was impatient and after several weeks asked the trainer, "Can we have a tournament?"
>
> The trainer told him, definitely not. The rooster was not ready. Yes, he was strong enough and knew many powerful combat techniques but his strength was empty, full of hot air. "He wants to fight all the time, is over excited and has no endurance."
>
> Several weeks later, the king again approached the trainer with the same question. Again the answer was he was not ready. "He's still too fierce, he still wants to fight all the time, even when he hears a rooster crowing in the next village, he becomes enraged and wants to engage in combat."
>
> The king waited, and gave the trainer an extra month and came to him again. The trainer said "Well, he no longer becomes enraged with passion, he remains calm and never seems to loose

> his temper. Actually, when you look at him you aren't really aware of his energy and strength. So the king continued to press the trainer, "Can we have a tournament?" The trainer finally answered "maybe." So on the day of the tournament all of the great fighting cocks were assembled and the contest began. But no rooster would come any where near the king's champion. They were all terrified of him and he never needed to fight.
>
> The king's champion had gone beyond his technical training. He possessed enormous energy, but it was inside of him. He never showed it. That way, his power stayed within himself, and the other roosters had no choice but to bow before his tranquil assurance and un-displayed strength.
>
> The true way of Budō is not through conflict. Actually the traditional practice of karate-dō has been greatly influenced by Bushidō (the way of the warrior). The secret of the sword is to never unsheathe it. Instead of killing an opponent, one must first kill themselves, their own mind. When we can accomplish this, we become much stronger, with harmony, harnessing our power and energy. We can then become a strong and positive human and avoid conflict (like the rooster).

This concept is so easily stated, but so very difficult to accomplish. It must start with practicing the physical techniques for many, many years. These techniques combined with our ki form powerful techniques through our breathing. The first two concepts, if practiced diligently will eventually lead you to seek out and discover the *shin*, the right attitude of mind. Another way to say this is to say that you begin to gain a sense of maturity and, therefore, can bring the *shin* of your soul to the surface to be sensed by all of those you encounter.

Perhaps this final chapter has become somewhat philosophical. True karate practice has some of these elements, but these elements will only become apparent after you have trained rigorously for many years.

I invite anyone who wishes to polish themselves through this noble martial art, to step forward and begin their training with a qualified instructor.

I think this small work should be punctuated by taking a quote from the *Bubishi*, the document which has become known as the bible of karate. Article fourteen states in part

> If everyone learned these methods there would be less violence. These methods are intended to foster peace and harmony, not violence. If you know someone with these special skills you should ask them to teach you. The rewards of training are immeasurable for those who remain diligent and follow the correct path. However, this does not apply to those of immoral character.
>
> When forced to fight, theory and technique are one in the same; victory depends upon who is better prepared. When engaging the adversary, respond instinctively. Movement must be fast and materialize without thought. Never underestimate your opponent, and be careful not to waste energy on unnecessary movement. If you recognize or create an opening, waste no time in taking advantage of it. Should he run, give chase but be prepared, expect the unexpected, and do not get distracted. You must evaluate everything when fighting....
>
> The more you train, the more you will know yourself..... Never underestimate any opponent, and be sure never to use any more force than is absolutely necessary to assure victory, lest you be defeated yourself.... These are the principles of ancient law.

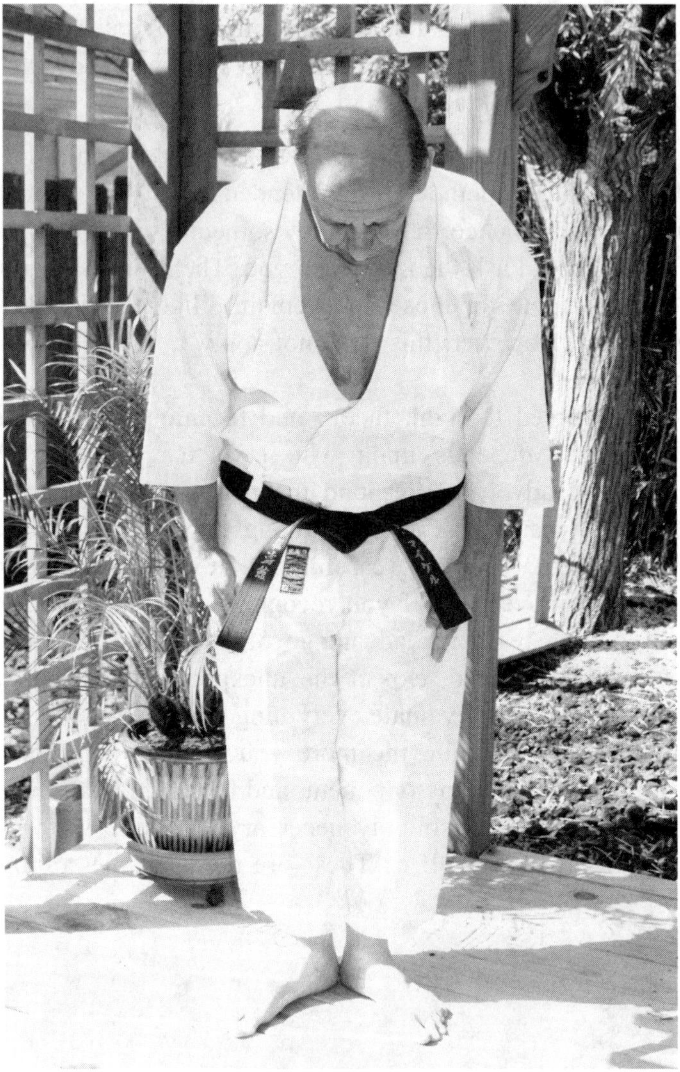

Figure 43: Rei.

[1] Don DePree, Shotokan Karate of America, *Relevance of Karate Practice.*
[2] Trevor Leggett, *A First Zen Reader*, p. 215
[3] *Ibid.*, p. 204.
[4] Taisen. Deshimaru, *The Zen Way to the Martial Arts*, p. 90
[5] *Ibid.*, p. 72.
[6] *Ibid.*, pp. 50-51.

Appendix

Back-Fist (Uraken)

The fist of this technique is made as explained in Chapter 4 on hand techniques. The technique, however, is quite different from the thrusting techniques described in Chapter 4. The striking portion of the hand is also different, as well as the motion of the hip.

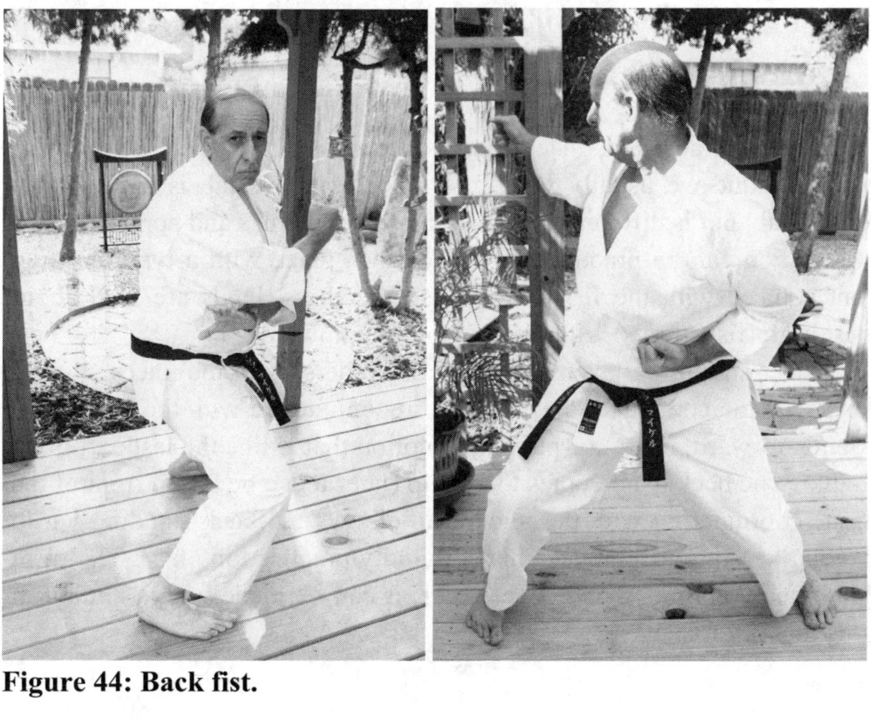

Figure 44: Back fist.

The uraken is made with a turning hip. The shoulder, arm, and fist become somewhat like the old combat weapon used by English knights in the Middle Ages. This weapon was a flail (sometimes known as a mace). Ohshima Sensei says that uraken "is one of the original, natural human movements.... We should all practice uraken until we are confident that, even against bigger, experienced opponents, we can make realistic kime (focused power) in our counterattacks."[1]

The basic practice of uraken is made from a kiba-dachi. The fist is made as described in Chapter 4. The attacking parts of the hand are knuckles of the index and middle finger. Try not to strike with other parts of the hand (other fingers, the wrist, or the flat portion). This can injure your hand and render the technique ineffective.

The power of this technique comes from a rotating hip. The arm motion is coupled with relaxed shoulders and upper body. The underarms are tightened at the moment of impact. Care should be taken not to straighten the elbow fully, which can lead to injury. (Refer to the photos.)

Jab (Maete)

Literally translated, maete means "front hand." When we practice this technique we usually refer to it as a jab. This jab is similar to a boxer's jab, but is different in terms of body dynamics and application.

The jab can be practiced by standing in place with a type of "high front stance" with the feet fairly close together. Hands are held about chest high (fists turned with fingers pointing upward).

Power should be taken out of the shoulders, with the knees slightly flexed. At the command, the front leg in conjunction with the front hand extends forward, making a punching motion that is like the last part of an oi-zuki. The back hand comes to the hip (later it can be left in front of the chest) coordinating with the underarm, elbow, and back standing leg to make a thrusting technique. This is initially practiced in place. The front side extends into a front stance. Later, it can be made with a sliding-in movement (yoriashi).

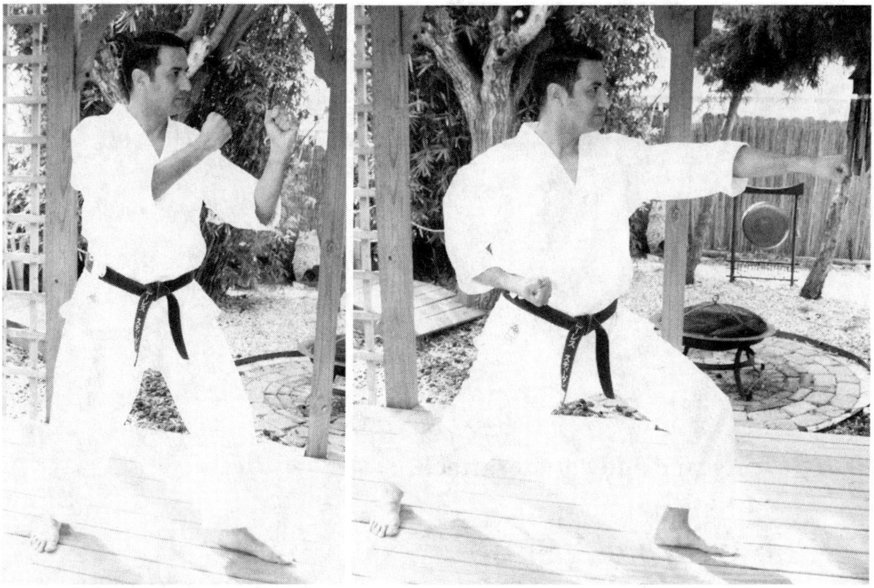

Figure 45: Jab.

Escaping Techniques (Torite)

Our practice of torite in an introductory class is a very brief introduction to the concepts of escaping from grabs of your body and clothes. This basic concept is introduced in conjunction with Heian Shodan.

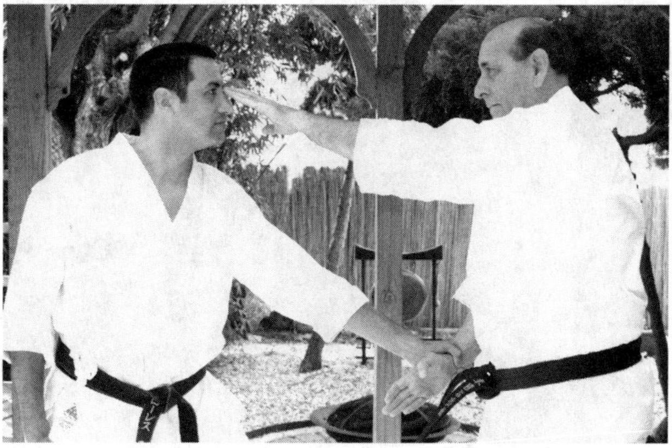

Figure 46: Escaping techniques.

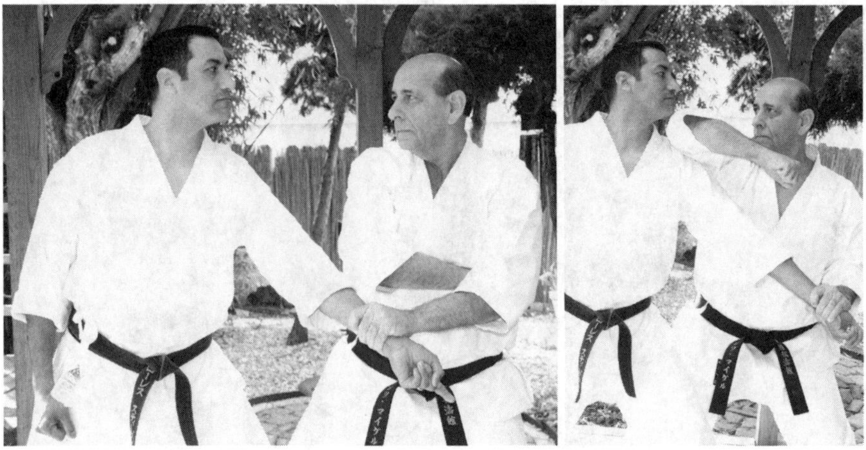

Figure 47: Escape and counterattack.

Elbow Strikes (Enpi)

The use of the elbow in self-defense situations is powerful and can be quite effective. The key to this technique is to be very close to the opponent and to connect your hip through your underarms and pulling hand.

The drawback is that it has a very short effective striking distance (basically from your shoulder to elbow).[2] Our practice in class will

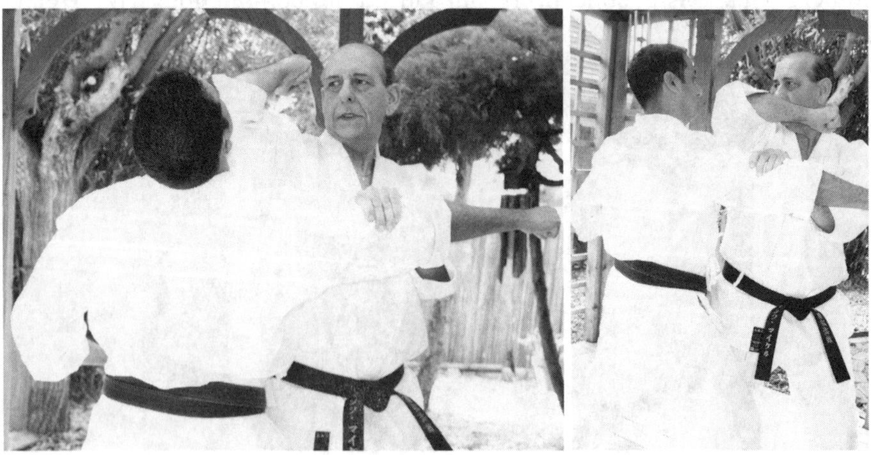

Figure 48: Elbow strikes.

consist of practicing the different angles of striking with the elbows (using a turning and straight hip): striking upward, downward, across laterally, backward up, straight back, or sideways.[3] A small form will be developed to practice the elbow strikes.

Footwork

Realistic movement for combat situations requires that you move freely without inhibitions. Training to move in different ways is one way to create the muscle memory necessary for efficient and effective movement in combat.

Several ways in which we will do this are moving forward in a front stance, moving backward in a back stance, moving forward by first stepping-up with the rear foot, making a sliding-in (yoriashi) movement with both legs while moving forward and back, and using a yoriashi movement in horse riding stance sideways and foreword.

Suggested Reading

Karate-Dō Kyōhan by Gichin Funakoshi, translated by Tsutomu Ohshima. Chapter 2. Fundamental Elements, pp. 17-21, Chapter 5. p. 235 (Methods of Practice).

---

[1] Tsutomu Ohshima, *Notes on Training*, p. 110.
[2] Tsutomu Ohshima, *Notes on Training*, p. 114
[3] Tom Muzila, Shotokan Karate of America.

Glossary

age-uke rising block
age-zuki rising punch
ashi waza kicks, leg techniques
ashibarai foot sweep
assume opposite direction kaette
assume stance kamaete
at ease yasume
back stance kōkutsu-dachi
back-fist strike uraken-uchi
barai (harai when used after other words) blocks
bari-bari continuous punches alternating hands
basic one-time sparring kihon ippon gumite
basic training kihon
begin hajime
belt obi
black belt rank dan
block uke, harai (changes to barai when used after other words)
bō staff
body tai
bottom-fist strike tetsui-uchi, tettsui-uchi
bow rei, lei
breathing center in lower abdomen tanden
brown belt rank kyū
Budō way of combat
Bushidō way of the warrior (samurai)
cat stance nekoashi-dachi

center and source of physical energy in lower abdomen hara
chūdan middle body, middle level
close-leg stance heisoku-dachi
combat form kata
continuous kicks renzoku-geri
continuous punches alternating hands bari-bari
continuous punching attacks renzoku-zuki, ren-zuki
continuous techniques renzoku waza
crescent kick mikazuki-geri
cross-arm block jūji-uke
dachi standing forms, stance
dan black belt rank
distance, timing, and other things between opponents ma
dō the way
dōjō training hall or place of training
double front kick nidan-geri
double punch morote-zuki
down block gedan-barai
elbow attack enpi (sometimes pronounced empi)
embusen line of movement in kata
empi (usually enpi) elbow attacks
enpi elbow attacks
escape techniques torite
feet together stance heisoku dachi
fist way quanfa (Chinese)
five-time sparring gohon gumite
flying front kick tobi-geri
flying side-thrust kick tobi-yokogeri
focus of techniques kime
foot edge sokutō
foot sweep ashibarai
forearm block ude-uke
fore-fist seiken
fore-knuckle fist hiraken
form kata
free one-time sparring jiyū-ippon gumite

free-style sparring jiyū kumite
front hand jab maete
front kick mae-geri
front kick with front leg maeashi-geri
front punch oi-zuki
front stance zenkutsu-dachi
front-thrust kick maeashi-kekomi
fudō-dachi immovable stance
fumikomi stamping kick
gasshuku special training (literally, to accommodate together)
gedan lower body
gedan-barai downward block
geri kick
get ready yōi
getting into the opponent irimi
gi training uniform
gohon gumite five-time sparring
gong fu Chinese martial art featuring empty hand techniques (literally, "hard work")
gumite sparring
gyaku-zuki reverse punch
hachiji-dachi open-leg stance
haitō ridge-hand
hajime begin
half-facing stance hanmi-dachi
hammer block tetsui-uke, tettsui-uke, uchikomi
hand te
hand techniques te waza
hanmi-dachi half-facing stance
hara center and source of physical energy in lower abdomen
harai blocks
head instructor shihan
heel kakato
heisoku-dachi close-leg stance, feet-together stance
hikite pulling hand
hiraken fore-knuckle fist

hizagashira kneecap
hook punch kagi-zuki
horse riding stance kiba-dachi
immovable stance fudō-dachi
inside forearm block ude-uke
instructor sensei
internal energy ki
ippon gumite one-time sparring
ippon-ken one-knuckle fist
irimi getting into the opponent
jab maete
jiyū kumite free-style
jiyū-ippon gumite free one-time sparring
jōdan upper body
jūji-uke cross-arm block
jumping-in attack tobikomi
kaette pivot, assume opposite direction
kagi-zuki hook punch
kakato heel
kamaete assume stance
karate-dō way of the empty hand
kata form
keiko gi training uniform
keri kick
ki internal energy
kiai spirit shout, union of energy, vocal expulsion of air
kiba-dachi horse riding stance
kibadachi-zuki punching with horse riding stance
kick keri (changes to geri when used after other words)
kihon basic training
kihon ippon gumite basic one-time sparring
kime focus of techniques, maximum effectiveness
kneecap hizagashira
knife hand block shutō-uke
knife-hand strike shutō-uchi
kōkutsu-dachi back stance

kumite sparring
kung fu Chinese martial art featuring empty hand techniques (literally, "hard work")
kyū white/brown belt rank
lei bow
level before black belt kyū
line of movement in kata embusen
lower body gedan
lunge punch oi-zuki
ma distance, timing, and other things between opponents
maeashi-geri front kick with front leg
maeashi-kekomi front-thrust kick
mae-geri front kick
maete front hand, jab
makiwara punching board
master instructor of an organization shihan
match shiai
mawashi-geri round kick
maximum effectiveness kime
meditation mokusō
middle body chūdan
middle finger/knuckle fist nakadaka-ken
middle level chūdan
mikazuki-geri crescent kick
mokusō meditation
morote-uke two-hand block
morote-zuki double punch
move into position kamaete
nagewaza throwing techniques
nakadaka-ken middle finger/knuckle fist
natural stance shizentai
nekoashi-dachi cat stance
nidan-geri double front kick
nihon-nukite two-finger spear-hand
nukite spear-hand
obi training uniform belt

oi-zuki front punch, lunge punch
one-knuckle fist ippon-ken
one-time sparring ippon gumite
open-leg stance hachiji-dachi
palm-heel block teishō-uke
palm-heel teishō
pivot kaette
pulling hand hikite
punch tsuki (zuki when used after other words)
punches te waza
punching board makiwara
punching with horse riding stance kibadachi-zuki
quanfa (Chinese) fist way
rank (black belt) dan
rank before black belt kyū
ready yoi
rear kick ushiro-geri
rei bow, salute
relax yasume
renzoku-geri continuous kicks
renzoku-waza continuous techniques
renzoku-zuki continuous punching attacks
ren-zuki continuous punching attacks
rest yasume
reverse punch gyaku-zuki
ridge-hand haitō
rising block age-uke
rising punch age-zuki
round kick mawashi-geri
salute rei, lei
sanbon gumite three-time sparring
seiken fore-fist
sensei instructor
shiai match
shihan head instructor/master instructor of an organization
shin spirit mind, soul-attitude

shizentai natural stance
shutō knife hand
shutō-uchi knife-hand strike
shutō-uke knife-hand block
side-thrust kick yokogeri-kekomi
side-up kick yokogeri-keage
sliding technique yoriashi
sokutō foot edge
soul-attitude shin
space between opponents ma
sparring kumite (often becomes gumite when used after other words)
spear-hand nukite
special training gasshuku
spirit mind shin
spirit shout kiai
staff bō
stamping kick fumikomi
standing forms tachikata (tachi changes to dachi when used after other words)
stop (remain ready) yame
striking techniques uchi waza
sword hand shutō
tachi standing forms
tachikata standing forms
tai body
tanden breathing center in lower abdomen
te hand
te waza punches, hand techniques
technique waza
teishō palm-heel
teishō-uke palm-heel block
tetsui-uchi (tettsui-uchi) bottom-fist strike
tetsui-uke (tettsui-uke) hammer block
three-time sparring sanbon gumite
throwing techniques nagewaza
thrust tsuki (changes to zuki when used after other words)

thrusting technique tsuki (zuki when used after other words)
tobi-geri flying front kick
tobikomi jumping-in attack
tobi-yokogeri flying side-thrust kick
torite escape techniques
training hall dōjō
training uniform belt obi
training uniform gi, keiko gi
tsuki thrust
turn in opposite direction kaette
two-finger spear-hand nihon-nukite
two-hand block morote-uke
uchi waza striking techniques
uchikomi hammer
ude-uke inside forearm block
uke block
uniform gi
union of energy kiai
upper body jōdan
upper level jōdan
uraken back fist strike
uraken-uchi back-fist strike
ushiro-geri rear kick
vocal expulsion of air kiai
way dō
way of combat Budō
way of the empty hand karate-dō
way of the warrior (samurai) Bushidō
waza technique
white belt rank kyū
yame stop (remain ready)
yasume rest, relax, at ease
yōi get ready
yokogeri-keage side-up kick
yokogeri-kekomi side-thrust kick
yoriashi sliding technique

zenkutsu-dachi front stance
zuki thrust, punch

Numbers

one	ichi (ee-chee)
two	ni (nee)
three	san (sahn)
four	shi (shee)
five	go (goh)
six	roku (roh-koo)
seven	shichi (shee-chee)
eight	hachi (hah chee)
nine	ku (koo)
ten	ju (joo)

Basic Commands

assume a position	kamaete
begin	hajime
bow	rei
meditate	mokusō
pivot	kaette
ready	yoi
rest	yasume
stop (remain ready)	yame

Test Questions

1. **What is the translation for "karate-dō"?**
   The way of the empty hand.
2. **Who is considered the father of modern karate?**
   Master Gichin Funakoshi.
3. **Name the three facets or major areas of karate practice.**
   Basics (kihon), forms (kata), sparring (kumite).
4. **Name the master text of karate-dō, authored by Master Gichin Funakoshi.**
   Karate-Dō Kyōhan: The Master Text.
5. **Name the individual who translated The Master Text.**
   Tsutomu Ohshima.
6. **What name(s) were used to describe the original indigenous Okinawan martial art?**
   Te, or bushi-no-te.
7. **List the three Okinawan cities that gave birth to the spread of karate.**
   Shuri, Naha, Tomari.
8. **Who were the two great karate masters who instructed Master Funakoshi?**
   Master Anko Itosu, Master Anko Azato.
9. **Who brought Shotokan Karate to the United States in 1955?**
   Tsutomu Ohshima.

10. Who created the system for training the Shaolin monks in China (520 AD)?
Bodhidarma (also known as Ta-Mo or Lao-tsu).

11. What was this system eventually called?
Gong fu (kung fu) or quanfa.

12. What is the *Bubishi*?
The bible of karate.

13. What year was karate first publicly introduced in Japan?
1922 by Gichin Funakoshi.

14. What was the original meaning of the word karate? What is the new meaning as revised by Master Funakoshi?
The original meaning was Chinese hand; the revised meaning is empty hand.

15. What is the meaning of the word "rei"?
Bow or salute (everything always begins and ends with rei).

16. What is a gi?
A training uniform.

17. What is mokusō?
Meditation.

18. What part of the anatomy generates the power for the karate practitioner's technique?
The powerful hips.

19. How many basic ways do we move our hips when we practice?
Three ways
1) straight (forward and back)
2) straight (side to side)
3) turning

20. How many basic stances do we have?
Seven basic stances.

21. Name the seven stances.
1) Hachiji-dachi (natural)

2) Zenkutsu-dachi (front)
3) Kōkutso-dachi (back)
4) Kiba-dachi (horse riding)
5) Nekoashi-dachi (cat)
6) Heisoku-dachi (feet together)
7) Fudō-dachi (immovable)

22. What is a hikite?
Pulling hand.

23. What is meant by waza?
Technique.

24. What is a kiai?
Spirit shout. The union of energy. Our internal energy expressed outwardly.

25. Name the different types of powers in karate.
1) Thrusting
2) Snapping
3) Swinging.

26. What are the basic blocks?
1) Gedan-barai (down block)
2) Ude-uke (inside forearm block)
3) Age-uke (rising up block)
4) Tetsui-uke (hammer block)
5) Shutō-uke (knife hand block)

27. Name the two basic punches or thrusting techniques.
1) Oi-zuki (front punch)
2) Gyaku-zuki (reverse punch)

28. Name the six basic kicking techniques.
1) Mae-geri (front kick)
2) Mawashi-geri (round kick)
3) Yokogeri-keage (side-up kick)
4) Yokogeri-kekomi (side-thrust kick)
5) Mikazuki-geri (crescent kick)
6) Fumikomi (stamping kick)

29. What is a kata?
A combat form with offensive and defensive techniques.

30. What is the embusen?
The line of movement for each kata.

31. Name the three cardinal points from Master Funakoshi for practicing katas.
1) Expansion and contraction
2) Slow and fast movements
3) Light and heavy application of strength

32. What is the meaning of Taikyoku?
First cause.

33. What is the meaning of Heian?
Peaceful mind.

34. What are the two distinct schools of katas described by Master Funakoshi in *Karate-Dō Kyōhan*?
1) Shōrin-ryu
2) Shōkei-ryu

35. What is the embusen for Taikyoku Shodan, Heian Shodan, and Heian Nidan?
I-embusen.

36. What do the terms, 1) yoi, 2) yame, and 3) yasume mean?
1) Ready
2) Stop (ending ready)
3) Rest, relax

37. How many katas are included in the *Karate-Dō Kyōhan* (including Ten No Kata)?
Nineteen katas.

38. The traditional Ways to self-improvement (dō) are said to contain two distinct wings. Name them.
1) Technical
2) Transcendence of technique

39. What is the name of the kata that is practiced for development of sparring (mainly one-time sparring)?
Ten No Kata.

40. What is meant by basic ippon gumite?
Basic one-time sparring.

41. What is meant by basic sanbon gumite?
Basic three-time sparring.

42. What is a dōjō?
Training hall or place of training.

43. What is the meaning of Bushidō?
The way of the warrior.

44. What is the *shin*?
Spirit mind, soul attitude.

45. What is the term for escaping techniques?
Torite.

46. Name the Japanese numbers 1-10.
1) Ichi
2) Ni
3) San
4) Shi
5) Go
6) Roku
7) Shichi
8) Hachi
9) Ku
10) Ju

47. Define the following terms: 1) kamaete, 2) hajime, 3) kaette.
1) Assume a stance
2) Begin
3) Pivot or assume the opposite direction

48. Define the word Shoto in Shotokan Karate.
Shoto means "pine waves," the sound that the wind made through the pine trees on Mount Torao.

49. Who was the founder or creator of the Naha-Te style of karate?
Master Kanryo Higashionna.

50. Who were the two masters who created 1) Goju-Ryu, and 2) Shito-Ryu?
1) Master Chojun Miyagi.
2) Master Kenwa Mabuni.

Bibliography

Books

Deshimaru, Taisen. *The Zen Way to the Martial Arts*. New York: E.P. Dutton, Inc. 1982.

Egami, Shigeru. *The Heart of Karate-Dō*. Tokyo, New York, San Francisco: Kodansha International, 1980.

Funakoshi, Gichin. (translated by Tsutomu Ohshima). *Karate-Dō Kyōhan: The Master Text*. Tokyo, New York, San Francisco: Kodansha International Ltd., 1973.

Funakoshi, Gichin. *Karate-Dō: My Way of Life*. Tokyo, New York, San Francisco: Kodansha International, 1975.

Funakoshi, Gichin. (translated by John Teramoto). *Karate-Dō Nyūmon*. Tokyo, New York: Kodansha International, 1988.

Funakoshi, Gichin. (translated by John Teramoto). *Karate Jutsu*. Tokyo, New York, London: Kodansha International, 2001.

Funakoshi, Gichin. (translated by John Teramoto). *The Twenty Guiding Principles of Karate*. Tokyo, New York, London: Kodansha International, 2003.

Herrigel, Eugen. (translated by R.F.C. Hull). *Zen in the Art of Archery*. New York: Vintage Books, 1953.

Kane, Lawrence and Wilder, Kris. *The Way of Kata*. Boston: YMAA Publication Center, Inc. 2005.

Leggett, Trevor. (compiled and translated). *A First Zen Reader*. Rutland Vermont, Tokyo: Charles E. Tuttle Company, 1960.

McCarthy, Patrick. (commentary and translation). *The Bible of Karate Bubishi*. Tokyo, Rutland, VT, Singapore: Tuttle Publishing, 1995.

Merton, Thomas. *Zen and the Birds of Appetite*. New York: New Directions, 1986.

Muzila, Tom. *Mental Karate: A Warrior's Guide*. Los Angeles: Empire Books, 2006.

Musashi, Miyamoto. (translated by Victor Harris). *A Book of Five Rings*. Woodstock, New York: Overlook Press, 1974.

Nitobe, Inazo (compiled and edited by Charles Lucas). *Bushidō: The Warrior's Code*. Burbank, CA: Ohara Publications Inc., 1979.

Ohshima, Tsutomu. *Notes on Training*. Ravensdale, WA: Pine Winds Press, 1998.

Roth, Jordan. *Black Belt Karate*. Rutland, VT, Tokyo, Japan: Charles E. Tuttle Co., 1974.

Schmeisser, Elmar T. *Channan: Heart of the Heians*. Ishikawa-Ken, Japan: Usagi Press, in cooperation with Trafford Publishing.

Suzuki, Daisetz T. *Zen and Japanese Culture*. Princeton: Princeton University Press. 1959.

Web Site

www.ska.org — Shotokan Karate of America

Documents

DePree, Don. *The Relevance of Karate to Everyday Life: A Collection of Practice Notes and Thoughts from Don DePree*. Shotokan Karate of America Inc, 1992, 1993, 1994.

Sagawa, Jim. *The Road to Irimi: Practice Notes from Jim Sagawa on the Ohshima Method for Practicing Shotokan Karate*. Shotokan Karate of America Inc., 2008.

Video / DVD

Muzila, Tom. *Shotokan Karate* Vols. 1-5. Lubbock, Texas: Black Belt Magazine Video, 1999.

About the Authors

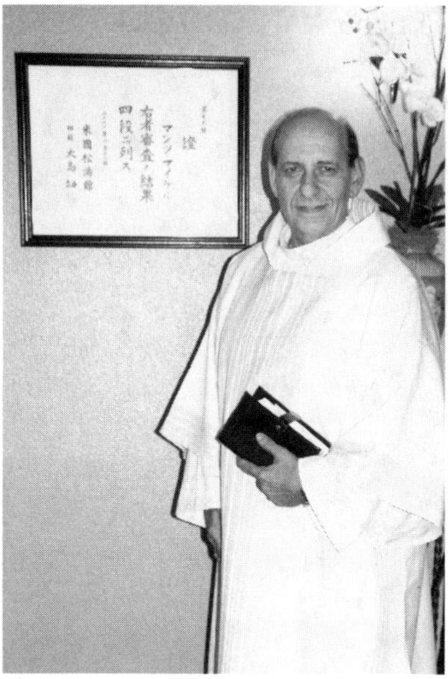

Michael Mantz is an adjunct professor in Kinesiology at Del Mar College and Texas A&M University — Corpus Christi, teaching college credit courses in karate. He also teaches karate for the Corpus Christi Independent School District's Collegiate High School Program.

He is a fourth degree (yodan) black belt in Tsutomu Ohshima's Shotokan Karate of America, training in traditional Karate for over 35 years.

Mr. Mantz is also an ordained Roman Catholic Deacon and currently serves as the Director for Deacons in the Diocese of Corpus Christi.

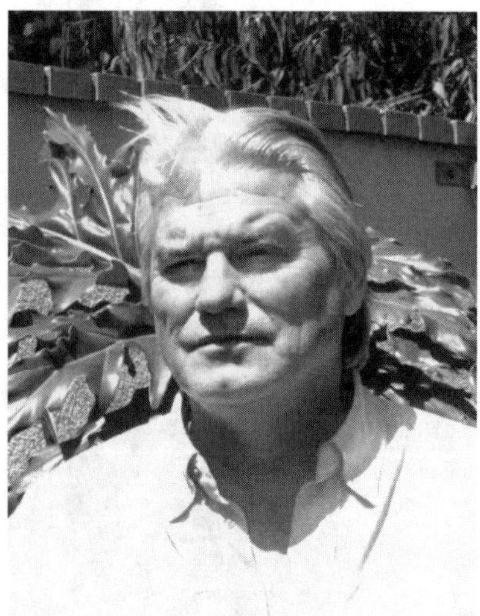

Tom Muzila has over 45 years of practicing and teaching martial arts and fitness conditioning.

He is a fifth degree (godan) black belt in Tsutomu Ohshima's Shotokan Karate of America. Tom has established several world marks and long endurance karate records.

He is a former US Army Special Forces (Green Berets) and a specialist in Optimum Peak Performance Mental States. Mr. Muzila is also a counter-terrorism specialist with over 30 years of professional body guarding experience. He has taught SWAT teams and elite military units. Tom has authored *Mental Karate: A Warrior's Guide*. You can visit Tom at his website www.tommuzila.com.